Gingivitis & Gum Disease A Fight to Keep My Teeth and Save My Life

Morgan G. Meyers Adams

MORGANS ALOHA EARTH CORPORATION

If you like the front cover design of my book as much as I do, you can order a tshirt version on my website, and support oral health awareness.

morgansbooksshirtsandmore.com

helphomelessanimalsinhawaii.org

A portion of all proceeds will go to my charity Help Homeless Animals in Hawaii, and other favorable charities.

DEDICATION

Dedicated to my dear son Max, he pushed me tirelessly, when I was exhausted. He took care of the house, our pets, and the cooking. So that I could work, write this book, and make this miracle happen.

Information provided in this book are accurate and current to the best of my knowledge, and resources, at the time that it was written. Many statements made are subject to change. There are no guarantees. I am offering my insight, advice, and opinions.

Table of Contents

INTRODUCTION

This story reflects my personal journey, it depicts my life, experiences, and how my pregnancy gingivitis at the age of nineteen, has now led to gum disease at the age of forty four. It has become a battle, to gain, and maintain, optimal oral health that I will be engaged in for a lifetime. Allow me to share what I have learned, and feel, to be the most valuable oral health care knowledge. I believe my own practiced tips, will make a positive impact in your life. Join me, defend yourself, keep your teeth, and save your life.

1
Silent Disease

There is a silent and deadly killer that lives in our mouths, and it is time for all of us to understand what this means, and to talk about the potential danger this bacteria may cause if ignored. It is insidious. You may not even know that you have it. It is a silent disease that will cause tooth decay and gum destruction, and there is no cure. Gum disease is irreversible. Only brushing, flossing and costly treatments are available if one can afford them to prevent further progression. I feel it is imperative to bring this topic more into the light. To raise the awareness level, by helping people to avoid this health hazard, or to identify the signs that it already exists, and give them the information that is necessary to fight it. Whether you have a healthy mouth, or may be one out of the possible eighty percent of our population that may have gingivitis, or a worse stage of periodontal gum disease. Some people may not even know that they have it. Everyone needs to understand why this type of bacteria is a potential killer, I am sharing all of the most important vital information that I have learned from my own experience, and diligent research. The tips that I share in this book could save your life. I have researched this subject extensively and have compiled a collection of what I felt to be the most pertinent facts, useful information, as well as a few of my own self-taught tips that I believe will be very helpful and necessary to fight this silent disease. You see, now that I know what I have learned, I have come to the conclusion that the bacteria living in our mouths is just as dangerous as fecal bacteria. But the germs that live in our mouths have a much slower process of harming our health. Basically though, it's like mouth poop. If you are not brushing and flossing before you go to bed, then you are sleeping with plaque poop in your mouth. How disgusting is that thought? Very, but that is exactly what it is like, so I hope to shock or scare you into brushing and flossing daily, most importantly at bedtime. I need to scare myself. I am picturing me with dentures, after losing all of my teeth. I will smack my toothless gums together trying to smile. I think about the damage that this plaque will do if it enters into any of my organs, like stroke or heart attack. This is the reality of it, and it is scary. Take the time to really think about this, and to find a deep soulful consciousness of how important it really is to be consistent with flossing every morning and most importantly every evening before bed. This is my battle, and I hope to help people swiftly comprehend something that took me far too long. When I began to really think about these germs turning into mouth poo, my brushing and flossing habits became consistent. When I voiced this opinion to my twenty four year old son, and a friend of mine, they soon became consistent with their flossing. So maybe this belief, as gross and weird as it sounds, might do the trick for you too, and make your brushing and flossing habits a daily occurrence. A majority of the people that I know either personally or from work could benefit from reading this book. They do what I used to, like not flossing consistently, if at all, and some occasionally will eat and then fall asleep without brushing their teeth. I tell them what I said to my son, and later I will give them a copy of this book, and that is the best that I can do to help them. Any kind of positive change can only come from within. I could not excuse myself with anymore reasons not to do it. I may think, oh I am just too tired, or I am in too much pain, and I will do it in the morning. When I begin to think like this now, I simply tell myself that I would be sleeping with poop in my mouth all night long. It is a disgusting thought, it is enough to make me get up from my daze and make my way to the sink to floss and brush. Why would anyone want to sleep with a mouth full of harmful bacteria that will stink like crap by the time you are finished sleeping. I have a very keen sense of smell, so it is possible that you may never have the experience that I had of smelling something similar to poop as I flossed my teeth after just a few days of not flossing. Gross. The deeper the pockets become around your teeth, the more crap that gets in between your teeth and gums. I used to make excuses and tell myself that I am going to do it later. I always felt like it was such a disgusting thing to do. Pulling the crud out from between all of my teeth, and then comes the blood with that horrible taste. Its gross, I particularly do not like to watch someone else floss, and if they are not doing it in the bathroom, I can get real disgusted by that. It is a minuscule amount of germ debris that you may not even see, but none the less it does come out of your mouth along with the floss that is being pulled out. So people please have the courtesy to do it over the sink. I remember one day I had a customer come in to the store where I work, he bought a bag of floss picks, while his wife looked around the store, he began to floss pick his teeth standing right there in front of my counter. I mean really, seriously, some people have no manners. I was inwardly horrified. I did not say anything to him because my new goal with customers is to make sure that I do not get in to any negative altercations with them. I do not have the time to do the damage control that is necessary when I stand up to rude or disturbed people. The first thing these people do when they are told something that they do not like is to get my name and to go make a complaint against me. Suffice it to say that I have learned. I am not capable of holding back the dangerous words that my mind is thinking. Sometimes the smartest thing to do is to do nothing. I simply just ignore all of my annoying customers, and their negative comments. My goal is to provide a professional service with courtesy, and that gets them out of my hair a lot quicker, even if it means putting up with their bad attitudes until they leave. If that does not work, then I will call security on them, and maybe they will come to help me, or not, I never know if they will really come, and it is never quickly. In this case I backed away from the counter to put more distance between us. It was really gross to watch a stranger standing right there in front of me while flossing potentially deadly germs out of his mouth.

Yes, potentially deadly germs. It is great that this man was flossing, but seriously, it is important that it should be done over the sink and in front of the mirror, and not in a public place in front of a stranger. I ask my loved ones to please stay in the bathroom when flossing. I do not want to sit at a table or on a couch where people floss the crap out from between their teeth. So people please have courtesy when flossing and be clean about it, and never go to sleep with poop in your mouth. There are many people that do this, and if you are one of them, then you need to stop right now. It is up to you to take what I say to heart, follow the tips, and make changes for your health and the span of your life. This is enlightenment towards better health. To understand that cavities and gum disease are caused by colonies of bacteria that continually coat the teeth with a sticky film called plaque. It collects and builds up at the gum line. If it is not brushed and flossed away, these bacteria break down sugars and starches in foods to produce acids that wear away the tooth enamel. The plaque hardens into tartar, an incrustation on the teeth, which can lead to gum inflammation or gum disease. A balanced diet provides vitamins, minerals, and other necessary nutrients for healthy teeth and gums. Fluoride produced naturally in foods is the best. Having it added to the water supply is another way to help reduce the rate of cavities by as much as fifty to sixty percent. The consensus of this opinion is based on the twenty nine studies done in one hundred and twelve countries. So there is research out there that seems to prove that fluoride does work.

My hygienist told me a story about a woman that kept coming back with new cavities until they made her a custom mouth piece that would hold the fluoride into her teeth. Then she stopped getting new cavities. But ultimately it is our habits that are going to make the most difference. If you have been taking care of your mouth and have healthy teeth and gums, then a big kudos to you. Keep it up for your lifetime. For the rest of us, transforming a bad habit into a good healthy habit is a difficult thing for the majority of us to do. Whether it may be with diet, exercise, or oral health care, switching our behaviors from negative, lazy, and unmindful patterns to positive awareness that leads us to change is a challenge for us all, and the utmost rewarding if we succeed.

2
Crazy Life

Let me entertain you for just a bit and tell you about the good and bad things of my crazy life, and many reasons I have to use as excuses to not floss. I have financial stress from the decline of tenants in my partnership commercial property that I own in Rapids City, South Dakota. Our building used to be full, and now we have many empty suites. So I work full time to compensate the loss of income. I am often busy with appointments, shopping, and running errands in the late morning to early afternoon before I go home and get ready for work. I drive forty five minutes to an hour depending on traffic at two in the afternoon. I work in resort retail on a sixty two acre resort and spa. I walk fifteen minutes from my car to the store with my loaded up backpack carrying snacks, drinks, dinner, cat food, meds, vinegar, and personal items. I walk and stand on stone and hard floors for eight hours, sitting for just a few minutes during my one break allowed. I may service anywhere from fifty to two hundred customers during my shift, doing the work of two people. Being a cashier is a difficult task alone, due to the fact that we accept guest charges as well as cash, credit cards, travel checks, and gift certificates. I may have a line of people for hours paying by guest charge, and that means printing out a total of six receipts between two computers, having the customer print last name, room number, and then signing the receipt. It has to be on three of the receipts, then stapled to the other three receipts and filed in three slots for each guest charge transaction. My coworkers use a carbon copy and line up each receipt in it, and ask them to fill it out. I can't take the snickering and comments for using such a ridiculous old school method, so I just have them fill out the first receipt to have at least one original copy, and then I fill out the other two receipts with last name and room number, and file all of the copies. Hundreds of guest charges per week when the hotel is full with corporate groups. People come in from all over the world, and if they do not speak English, we play charades until we can come to an understanding, or not. I stock the store, keeping the shelves filled. From drinks in the cooler, chips, snacks, cigarettes, alcohol, tee shirts, resort wear, jewelry, souvenirs, medicines and more. All inventory delivered will have to be checked in, priced, put out, and stored. The tee shirts must be folded perfectly with papers, and size label stickers put on each shirt. I sweep, mop, dust shelves, clean glass, doors, and keep the store clean. I stay busy attending to customers, answering questions, phones, and helping people pick out gifts, because some of my customers do not have a clue as to what they want to buy. Most people are nice and polite, but others can be difficult and mean, or just plain crazy. Then add alcohol or whatever pill they are on to the equation, and now they are dangerous. One night as I was leaving, I had to run away and hide from a mean drunken man that looked like a Viking. Security already been alerted by the bar that he was trouble, and came into my shop looking for him. I said I would call them if I see him. Well later I did see this man, I called security, and they did not come. I was on my own trying to leave to go home. This guy was scary as he was slurring curse words at me. He wanted for me to stop and talk to him or he was going to slap me. So I ran like a player on the defense team. There was a night when I got into a fight with an older teenage boy who was with a group of young men in the parking lot. I caught him vandalizing the cats feeding station and chasing all of the cats. I lost my temper and I screamed so loud and with so much anger, that they left, and I reported them to security. Not that it helped me any. I feel like I deal with a lot of negativity that comes at me from different places on an almost daily basis. All I desire in my life, and of myself, is to be a positive person and to be surrounded by others like me. So this job is becoming more and more stressful for me, being that I have to first calm down, process, release, and shake off so much negativity all of the time. It wears me down. I am so grateful for all of the truly kind people that I do encounter, because they make up for the bad ones. Kind people give me those rare good days, and I really do appreciate them. I sell around forty thousand dollars or more of merchandise a month. That is a lot of work for just one person to do in a busy resort gift shop. These years have given me experience and wisdom, having contact with so many people from all around the world has been very interesting to say the least. I feel that I really know the

good and the bad in all types of people. I am aware of
the games the cons, drunks, and trouble makers play. I
will close the store at ten pm, file all guest charges,
fold all shirts, fill the cooler, chips, and do banking
from the day and night shift. Record and balance the
cash, credit cards, guest charges, gift certificates, and
travel checks. Make a deposit, and get the four
hundred starting bank ready in the drawer for the
morning shift. Clean the glass, lock up, and then feed
nearly sixty cats that live on the grounds. I have seven
cats, and six kittens that I feed nearby, then it's a
fifteen minute walk to my car, taking the underground
tunnel to stop at the Finance Department and drop off
all of my guest charges. Some nights I may have
worked so hard, each step to the car hurts with
inflammation throughout my entire body, especially in
my knees. My left knee swells up larger than the size
of my right knee. I had Osgood-Schlatter disease in the
left knee as a kid, and will forever have problems with
it. I have osteoarthritis, which is a painful joint
disease, a lumbar degenerative disc in my back, carpal
tunnel in my right hand and arm, and the holes that my
nerves pass through in my neck have narrowed
causing pain from my neck down to my hands. When
my arthritis and exhaustion feels severe, inflammation
and bumps will swell up on my eye with pain equal to
that of a mean bug bite. My work has brought me pain
that I should not have felt until my older years, but I
would not trade it for a nine to five desk job. I would
become a butter ball, putting me more at risk for heart
attack and stroke. I am doing what I want to do if I am

going to have to work for someone other than myself. I am working hard at moving forward with my life, to succeed as an author, writing about my experiences in life, travel, and work. Immersing in philanthropy, helping animals and children are my passions, and gives great purpose to my life. I put tremendous effort into being an angel for cats, giving my love, time, and money to care for homeless cats. There is a feral cat organization in Hawaii, and this charity has helped spay and neuter almost forty thousand cats as of just the last time I heard the numbers. I am very grateful for their help, and the protection of a law they got passed that makes it illegal for anyone to harm or harass a feral cat or their feeder. Upon reaching my car, I will drive around the resort parking lot and feed fifty or more cats that live in two separate colonies. I would say that half of them are feral, some born and raised on the property, while the other half were formerly owned and abandoned or lost. Some of the cats are wild and tiger like, and I have to be careful around them. The others are sweet, very affectionate, following me around, and want me to stay with them. I feel sad when I have to leave them. I care for them two to four times a week, depending on other volunteers and their schedules. Giving them food, water, medicine, and trying to treat their wounds without them clawing or biting me. Usually their wounds are from fighting among each other or with the mongoose. I try to trap and deliver sick and dying cats to the Humane Society. I try to trap and deliver healthy cats to free clinics for spaying and neutering, and release them back into their environment. It is hard to trap cats, and sometimes the ones I need to go into the traps will avoid them, and then I am not able to help them. There is a dedicated woman that works at this resort and does most of the trapping, I am very grateful for her. Twice a month I will scrub algae out of the water dishes with vinegar and keep them clean. Whenever able to, I deliver food and water to cats that people abandon in lava fields. It angers me that people do this with their unwanted pets. There is no water, no birds, just lava desert, life is scarce, only a few rats, shrubs and thorny trees. Not a good place for any animal to be, and certainly not a domesticated one. I have set up six food and water stations so far. I make the difference between life and death for these cats. If they go more than two days without food, they could develop fatty liver disease, which may result in death. I cherish all animals, it does not matter if its dogs, goats, horses, birds, etc., whatever the situation is going to be, to help whenever present is my only choice. There is a huge over population of homeless cats on these islands. They need help from us humans. We owe it to them, for it was the irresponsibility of humans that caused this sadness, and it feels really good to make a positive difference in their lives. I usually arrive home by midnight, with a young adult son, four cats, and one dog to greet me. It will be an hour before I shower and brush my teeth. Later I may need to eat in order to sleep. I brush and floss my teeth now after eating and before sleeping. But there are still nights that I may feel dizzy, like my knees are going to buckle, and at that point flossing is not an option. I just want to make it through the brushing and fall in to bed. Upon waking I will brush and floss to make up for it, and since I do not eat breakfast for an hour after waking, my gums have time to stop stinging from flossing, and to allow the fluoride I use to do its job before I eat or drink anything. No doubt I need to continue to improve with my priority of flossing and to have no excuses for whatever level of pain and exhaustion I may be feeling. Now you can see how difficult it might be from the picture that I portray of my life, that there are many reasons to get in the way of caring for my overall health. You may be able to relate, on some level or another, life gets in the way of taking care of our own health. How do we muster up the time and energy for it? I should be excused for allowing my teeth and gums to rot right? Wrong, there is no excuse. I do not want to be living with rotten teeth and gums. No way! There are only two options, spend time and money now, or spend a whole lot of money and time later, or I just lose all of my teeth. When I think of the money, pain, and time that I could have saved had I cared for my mouth properly, it makes me want to kick myself hard in the butt. All I can do now is strive to make positive changes, a difficult challenge being that I work five days a week with two split days off. I no longer have time or energy for dating at this point in my life, did a lot of that in my earlier years, so I will worry about finding a companion in the near future. Currently I have reached a point of being burned out physically and emotionally. I rest whenever I am able to, take vitamins, supplements, eat healthy, drink water, brush, floss, and pray each day for more strength to come through my faith.

3
Insidious

This is a sneaky disease and most people are not aware it exists within them. The types of bacteria can vary from person to person. Some types are more associated with aggressive gum disease. When the bacteria have accumulated where the gums meet the teeth, it forms a ditch or a sulcus. It becomes periodontal, like what I have, and that is why they call it Periodontal Gum Disease. The spaces go all the way around the tooth like a moat around a castle. When the gums detach from the teeth and form pockets with a depth that is deeper than three millimeters, there is no chance of a person treating their own gum disease. The untreatable gum disease then spreads into the underlying bone which supports the teeth. If not treated early enough, the person will lose their teeth and their body is flooded by diseased biological molecules, which were produced by the gum tissues. Once gums have detached from the teeth forming pockets, food particles get in there, and the gum line becomes sensitive. I will rinse and swish warm water around my mouth to remove these particles, and if possible, brush and floss after every meal. Just brushing is not enough. If the food is left in between the teeth, and in these pockets for any length of time, it increases the inflammation, promotes bacteria growth, accumulates plaque, and the pockets will become deeper. I suggest using warm water because it helps break up and remove more food particles and germs. You should never drink or eat anything upon awakening in the morning until you have brushed your teeth and tongue first. Or at least swish and gargle with warm water, and preferably with sea salt. This will prevent the chance of getting sick from washing the dead cells, and bacteria into your intestines and stomach. Somehow I knew this even before I read it in a health article. All of my life I have rinsed and gargled, or brushed my teeth every morning before drinking or eating anything. It is just as important to clean the tongue after brushing the teeth. Always rinse out the brush first, then apply a small dab of toothpaste in the mouth, add a little warm water to swish it around, and brush the tongue all over, going as far back as you can without gagging yourself. Start in the back and brush forward. Brush the top of your mouth, and also the cheeks. This will eliminate bad breath odors, and prevent inflammation of the tongue caused by debris, bacteria, and dead cells. A white coating on the tongue is an indicator that you have an inflamed tongue, or an infection, and should be cleaned and treated right away. This infection is called Tongue Thrush, which occurs when fungus accumulates on the tongue and causes patches of white legions. The legions may be painful or bleed, try not to touch, because this will only make them worse. They can be found on your tongue, gums, tonsils or roof of your mouth. Thrush is more common in nursing babies, but adults can also get this condition. Especially for those who use inhaled corticosteroids and adults with weak immune systems. This yeast infection is called Candida, normally living in our bodies, it is not limited to the mouth, and can occur in other parts of the body as well. Illness, stress, medications, smoking, and dry mouth contribute to the yeast growth. Sugar and foods that contain yeast like bread, crackers, beer, and wine are also participating factors to disturbing the balance of this fungus, and it growing out of control. Antifungal medications can be described by your doctor. I successfully treated my own mild case of candida overgrowth in my body by taking daily probiotics and a teaspoon of organic unrefined pure coconut oil. The presence of candida infection can be a symptom of other medical problems, so seek care from a medical doctor as well. Lesions in your mouth could indicate oral cancer, and ulcers could mean high stress. A healthy tongue should have a pinkish color. Basically, a healthy mouth should look pink in the gums, tongue, and cheeks. Get healthy and be pink. If you are someone that gags too much when brushing your tongue, I suggest that you brush your teeth while you are in the shower to prevent that feeling. Open your mouth and let the water run down your tongue, and at the same time, take your toothbrush and swipe it from the back to the front until it is all clean. This really helps, and you will have a much cleaner mouth from the pressure of the water running into your mouth. I almost always brush during my showers, and my mouth feels a lot cleaner, and I prefer to swish the paste around my mouth with water before brushing. I have stopped chewing gum and candy. They are two of the worst things that you can put in your mouth. Instead I always carry a tube of toothpaste with me with fluoride or antibacterial ingredients. It is a smart way for me to keep my breath fresh in between brushing. I put a tiny dab of it in my mouth with a small amount of warm water if possible, swish it all around and through the teeth and gums before spitting it out. One important thing to remember is to expectorate when flossing, brushing, or rinsing. Spit out the germs and medicine from the mouth, throat, and lungs. Do not ever swallow. I highly recommend mixing a cup of warm water with sea salt for a soothing and refreshing mouth rinse. It kills germs, and will provide immediate relief of discomfort due to inflammation or flossing. Baking soda with warm water works well too. If you are going to use a mouthwash, look for more natural ones with no alcohol, since they can dry out your mouth and kill the natural antibodies in your saliva that fights germs, and help keep your mouth healthy and hydrated. Keep your toothbrush clean and stored in a sanitary place away from the toilet, where it can dry. A study proved that fecal bacteria can spread in the air when flushing the toilet, and was found on peoples toothbrushes. Keep a small bottle of dish soap near sink and rub a small dab of it on your toothbrush, rub the bristles and hold it under the tap to rinse with warm water at the same time, and then hold it under hot water for a few seconds to kill any remaining germs. Don't forget to cool it down with cool water before putting the toothbrush in your mouth. Clean your toothbrush before and after each use. There are some fancy products out there that will kill germs on toothbrushes if that's your kind of thing, but not necessary as long as you are cleaning them with soap on a daily basis. This will eliminate the transfer of nasty germs going back into your mouth. Replace the brush after two to three months. If you get sick, wash it extra good daily, and then replace your brush as soon as you are getting better. The best system is to rinse your mouth out first with warm water, brush, floss, and then brush away any food particles that have been dislodged from flossing. Slide your floss up and down, like a forward C, then a backward C, and slide it back and forth through each side of your tooth and gum. Brush in large circles first making your toothpaste foamy, then in smaller circles around the gum line. Not too hard or you could brush away gum tissue permanently. Hold toothbrush at an angle facing up for the top teeth and gum line, and then at a downward angle for the lower teeth and gum line. As a reminder, remember to brush the top of the mouth and cheeks. Rinse toothbrush and mouth, add another dab of toothpaste, and do another sweep around the mouth, then brush tongue really well. Rinse, gargle, and expectorate. This whole process of flossing and brushing takes me about five to ten minutes, depending on how much time I have. Use toothpastes with fluoride, antigingivitis, antibacterial triclosan, or prescription fluoride toothpaste. I use all of these. Triclosan is the key active ingredient used in Colgate Total Protection. I have heard that triclosan in soaps will pass in to our blood streams through our pores, damaging our systems natural balance of hormones. I wanted to research and learn what I could about it, and I was surprised at what I found. In 1997, the FDA reviewed extensive data on triclosan in Colgate Total toothpaste. The evidence showed that triclosan in this product was effective in the prevention of gingivitis. The agency does not have any evidence that triclosan in soap and body washes provides any added benefit than plain soap and water. Animal studies have shown that triclosan changes hormone regulation. But effects on animals do not predict effects on humans, and it is not currently known to be dangerous to humans. FDA is active in an ongoing scientific regulatory review of this ingredient. Just like with any chemical, we should not over expose ourselves to this ingredient. I use it because with my job, I need to use something that will fight the germs in my mouth for long periods of time.

4
Effects of Stress

Let me travel back in time for a moment. I remember getting my first cavities and having fillings put in around the time I was in grade school. I did see a dentist and hygienist on occasion, but never on a regular basis. I did not grow up with a mother or a father there to make sure I had brushed my teeth, and that I do not eat or drink anything after brushing other than water at bedtime. In fact it was quite the opposite, my father would have all night parties, and sometimes dinner would be anywhere between midnight and one in the morning. I would wake up and eat and then go right back to sleep without brushing. This was the beginning of a terrible habit that stayed with me for years. I paid more attention to keeping my lips soft and moisturized. One time when they were chapped my father told me to put some lip balm on, because they looked like an old ladies butt. Yeah that stayed with me forever, I am obsessed with keeping my lips soft. Instead I wish he would have told me to brush and floss my teeth, and that my breath stinks like an old ladies butt. I would have brushed and flossed all the time. Forgive me if you are an elderly lady reading this, no disrespect intended. My father had a sick sense of humor. I worded that nicely compared to his version. It was not an ideal life for me growing up, in some ways it was good, and in other ways it was sad. I moved around a lot as a child, between California,

Colorado, and Oregon. In my opinion these are definitely some of the best states to grow up in. I lived with friends of my dad's, my dad's girlfriends parents, or my aunt for three years before returning to my father in Colorado beginning of fifth grade. By the middle of eighth grade, my father was growing more unstable. The neglect, emotional, and physical abuse that I suffered resulted in the state taking custody of me. I lived in two foster homes and a county youth home within that one year's time before settling in with a former girlfriend of my father's, who at times worked for him doing secretarial tasks. I was finishing High School in Durango, Colorado, at the age of seventeen, and my estranged mother came to town and surprised me with an invite and tickets to come live with her in Maui, Hawaii. I talked mom into paying for my best friend Monica to come with me, since she was begging for me to not leave her in Durango. Then she died in Maui, just one year later, in a tragic car accident on Maui's most dangerous Hana highway. During that time I became pregnant and married, and less than two years later I left my husband and got a divorce. Those were very difficult times, from losing my best friend, to dealing with the heavy partying lifestyle that both my husband and my mother were engaged in. I became a young single mother with a special needs child. Oh, and the headaches that I got from almost every guy that I ever dated as a single mom certainly did not help. Stress has wreaked havoc in my life. As a child my son was diagnosed with ADHD, and as he grew there were apparent signs of mild OCD. These disorders are found in other family members on both sides, including me and his father. My son Max did not have a chance at escaping it, plus being born a preemie, I am really grateful that he has grown into such a wonderful person, and he is always evolving in positive form like me. I moved us to the Caribbean when my son was seventeen, seeking new and exciting experiences for both of us to grow upon. And we did. But the power and water company of Roatan Island went bankrupt shortly after we moved there. We went through hours each day without electricity and water, and after three months of no improvement I sent him to live with his father in Hawaii. His dad had cleaned up his act, and it was good for my son to get to know his father and family that lived in Hawaii. I returned to Hawaii six months later, and started working all of the time. Three years later my son moved back in with me, and not a moment too soon, for I discovered he was wound up as tight as a drum. He really needed to learn to relax, and focus on healthier interests, and improve his skills. Those signs of mild autism, or obsessive compulsions were more severe, and obvious to me. I educated myself by reading hours of online articles on the complete spectrum of autism. We worked hard together for positive behavior change, and to only have positive influences in both of our lives. We needed to be surrounded by compassionate, and understanding people. We had fun going to the farmers market, beach, and church together. We were baptized, that was a glorious day that we will never forget. My son is

doing marvelous and has surpassed my hopes or
expectations. I can say that he is doing better than
most adults I know. He has a maintenance job with a
reef teach program at a beach park. Rides his bike six
miles daily going to and from work. He takes care of
our pets, walking the dog twice a day, cleans the house
and yard, does the laundry, cooks, and has grown into
a fine young man whom I am very proud of. He has
healthy teeth and gums, drinks only water, no
smoking, eats very little sweets, brushes, and flosses
daily. Now that they are seeing a correlation between
gum disease and low birth weights, I wonder if this
could have been a participating factor in the case of
my son being born a preemie. Possibly. But most
likely not, because at that time I was not in any stage
of gum disease, I only had gingivitis. There were many
other factors involved such as stress and genetics. And
if stress is a contributing factor in gum disease, I am
sure it did a real number on me. I do know that when I
was pregnant it was the first time that I had ever heard
of having gingivitis. The changes in a pregnant
woman's hormone levels can increase her chance of
getting gum diseases. The milder form of gum disease
called pregnancy gingivitis can be controlled and most
likely would only be a small contributing factor in
delivering premature, or having a low birth weight
baby. My mother had miscarried a few pregnancies
after I was born. She had periodontal gum disease, I do
not know at what stage, but I do know that she had
problems with her teeth and had dental work done
periodically throughout her life. Drugs, alcohol,

smoking, and stress are all contributing factors in the rapid decay of my mother's gums, teeth, and health. At the age of fifty three, she suffered a stroke, and died within a month's time. Doctors say she had advanced liver cancer, and that was likely the cause for her stroke. But could her gum disease have played a part in her death as well? Possibly. There are some people who may have been born with genetically reduced resistance to gum disease. I do not know very much health information about my father, I only know that he did not take care of his health, lived hard, that he drank the hard stuff, did drugs, and died from ruptured ulcers at the age of forty nine. I just know that I fall into that category of people although I have never had any genetic testing for low gum disease resistance. Family profiling can be done to reconstruct a history of gum disease resistance. It is called a Clinical Disease Severity Aggressiveness Projection. I found it very interesting to learn that genetics and stress are participating culprits in gum disease. I can see how stress can affect our whole being, no matter what the situation might be, it drains us, and in result we do not take the best care of ourselves. Stress can influence our immune system. Our immune system is defined as a complex system of cells, organs and tissues that protect the body from bacteria, viruses and microorganisms that try to invade it. Stress suppresses immune system function, over time the immune system does not adapt but instead continues to wear away. Instead of protecting the body, it will begin to harm it. Stress and its effects on the immune system have been linked to cancer, AIDS and other autoimmune disorders. When the immune system has been worn down, it is not strong enough to fight off any dangerous bacteria that might be living in our bodies and mouths. The way stress affects the immune system is complicated but explained well in many health books, newsletters, and articles. One article, states that stress produces a hormone in the body called cortisol. The brain recognizes cortisol as the fight or flight hormone, when it is produced, other body functions are halted until the stressful situation has passed. This is the body's way of taking care of an immediate emergency. The immune system also receives signals to slow down while cortisol does its job. But with chronic stress, however, the immune system stays in low gear, leaving the body vulnerable to infection and disease. Common illnesses brought on or worsened by stress are cardiovascular disease, digestive problems, skin conditions, and poor memory function. The real problem is our failure to balance stress with intermittent rest. Push the body too hard for too long and you will have chronic stress, the result will indeed be burnout and breakdown. But subject the body to insufficient stress, and it will weaken and progressively decline. We actually need a small amount of stress. Few of us will not have pushed ourselves nearly hard enough to realize our potential, nor do we rest, sleep, and renew nearly as deeply or for as long as we should. Scientists have proven through their research that there is a correlation between illness, the immune system, and gum disease.

Diabetes can contribute to gum disease and research shows that gum disease can contribute to diabetes. A pregnant woman who is diabetic should make a periodontics appointment as soon as possible, for a thorough exam and care. Smoking, medications, dry mouth, calcium deficiencies and lifestyle are the contributing factors. Not brushing and flossing after meals, and before sleeping gives this bacteria a chance to breed and spread like destructive wildfires in the mouth. These microorganisms are like a rotten treacherous army in the mouth, and this is how we all need to think of them. I am in a battle, and this has become war. I am in a fight to keep my teeth, and save my life. But how did I get to this abysmal place of stage two of gum disease. Where my gums have begun to peel away from my teeth, leaving pockets, and becoming periodontal. Where more food and bio film plaque can settle in. I never paid that much attention to the inside of my mouth, and that was a big mistake. Now I look in the mirror every day and open my mouth wide to look at both front and the back side of my teeth and gums. Now I know how they are supposed to look. I literally have watched the gums slightly adhere themselves back around my teeth. I can see the pockets shrinking just a bit, especially on the inside of my bottom front teeth. But they have not closed up all the way, and it is possible that they never will. It seems that I am keeping this disease at bay, not allowing it to progress any further. I am treating it as aggressively as I can within my budget. If money was not an obstacle for me, I would be doing a lot more treatments with my hygienist and would have my fillings done right now. It has been five months now since my last visit, two months past the date that I was supposed to have another cleaning done.

5
Financial Priorities

Much of my extra money has been spent on the care of my pets because their health is important to me as well. Some people will think that is crazy. Others who can relate to that kind of selfless sacrifice and love for their pets will understand. Two of my cats have gingivitis and need cleanings as well to keep the plaque from getting in to their arteries or organs, and resulting in death just like humans. One cat is almost sixteen and because of her age and declining kidney function, it would be a risky procedure for her. But she really needs it, and to have some teeth pulled. Money is an obstacle, and without treatment, it will not get better on its own, only worse. I spend what I can afford to care for their health, but dental cleanings for my pets is just as costly as it is for me, so therefore they will have to wait until I can pay for their dental cleanings after mine. As for me, all this time between my dental cleanings has given the plaque a chance to build up again. I have scheduled an appointment for two weeks from now, and this time I can afford laser treatment as an extra option after the cleaning. It keeps plaque away for a longer period of time. I need that. When I think back in time, I remember my first real awareness with these germs began after I had my son, at the age of nineteen. During that time I started to see a new dentist and hygienist in Maui. They told me I had gingivitis, the early signs of periodontal disease, it was then that I remembered being told that I had gingivitis when I was pregnant. I did not have the oral health education or mindset to completely understand the real dangers of this living source growing in my mouth. There was not nearly as much research and information available back then either. Over the years I needed to have fillings and root canals, and I was seeing different dentists and hygienists on the island depending on where I lived at the time. I do not remember gum disease being brought to my attention again, only that I had this thing called gingivitis. Later around my early thirties I was living in Clearwater Beach, Florida, and I found a new dentist and hygienist that was a husband and wife team. They were a very nice couple, and seemed to be very good at what they do. Like most of us have had at one time or another, they had some very stressful family issues going on. I had asked them about the new groove lines that ran along my top two front teeth and gum line, I was told that it was probably acid erosion from sucking on citrus fruits, or that possibly could be the results of taking a certain antibiotic when I was a kid. Well that was partly true, I do have acid erosion since I have always loved to eat fruits, and that can do a lot of permanent damage to the enamel. Acids strip enamel from teeth. My grooves were also a direct result from my shrinking gum line due to my gum disease. Then in 2006 I moved off the Gulf coast of Florida, and went inland to a town called Hudson, near Newport Richey, which is where I found a very good dental office. I did not have insurance, but I had the cash available to take care of cleanings, and I needed more fillings. By this time all of my old unsafe mercury metal fillings have been removed and replaced with the new white resin that is now available, it matches your teeth, and I recommend paying the extra money for it. Then be careful after the work is done to not chip them by avoiding ice, hard veggies, candy, or anything that could cause a chip, and cost you more money. They also told me I had gingivitis, and gave me my first prescription fluoride toothpaste. It's stronger at fighting off plaque and cavities. It is a must have for my oral health care routine now. You definitely need to get this if you have gingivitis or any stage of gum disease. Later I spent almost a year living on Roatan Isle, Honduras, where the power company went bankrupt, half of every day or night we would be without power and running water. During the nine months that I lived and worked there, I did not seek out any local dentists, too scary. I was told it would be better to make a trip to the mainland of Honduras for quality dental care. I was still not using floss, even after being told to by my hygienist in Florida. Partly due to the fact that I still did not fully comprehend that it would make all of the difference in the health of my gums, and partly due to my mild OCD disorder, and how it was holding me back from flossing just because I did not like to do it. If that makes any sense. I have always brushed three to four times a day, but living on Roatan without power and water much of the time, I could only get in two brushings a day. That quickly led my gingivitis to progress to gum disease. I moved

back to Hawaii in September of 2007. I established
health care through my employer, but kept my costs
down by choosing one network, which provided only
one dental office within that network. So I made the
appointment, and went in for an exam, x-rays, and
cleaning. So far so good, and then the doctor came in.
He examined me, and did a lot of talking with the
women assistants in the room, making me feel like he
was not really paying attention to me or to what he
was doing. I asked him some questions, I wanted to
know the difference between Veneers and Lumineers,
and what option he thought would be best for my
teeth. He told me that his assistants will answer my
questions, as he exited the room. On top of that, the
office workers kept making mistakes, or forgetting to
do the things they told me they were going to do. I
never did return. That was a mistake I regret, I really
should have at least gone to get my teeth cleaned
again. One year later I could afford to upgrade my
insurance, which allowed me to see any participating
doctor of my choice. I live on the Big Island of
Hawaii, and it is much like being in another country.
My options are limited because as I discovered in
Kailua Kona town, there was only a couple of good
participating doctors and dentists available. My town
needs more doctors of all types.

6
Obtainable Options

So there are two very important factors here regarding the health of your mouth. One is money, oral health care is very expensive, and without insurance it is almost unobtainable for anyone not wealthy. With insurance it is still going to cost the copay. The other is finding the best dentist possible. Important things that I look for are state of the art equipment and procedures. Knowledgeable, caring, soothing and competent manners of the doctor, hygienist, and the assistants. A clean bathroom and comfortable office space are nice too. Are the office staff helpful and friendly, because we all know how terrible we all feel when we have to go visit the dentist, and it can make all the difference if they can make us feel a bit more comfortable. Soothe are nerves and our moods from the moment we enter the office. In the end of 2010, I chose an office that sounded like what I was looking for, and I got lucky because it was only two miles away from my home. Another husband and wife team. It has been a positive experience with them so far. I have not had any work done as of yet with the doctor other than my exams, but they went very well, he took his time with me, asking a lot of questions, and very thorough. Checking my jaw alignment, since I clench sometimes when sleeping from stress, this is called TMJ. He recommends making a molded mouth piece for me to where at night. I am going to pass on this for now. I do not feel that I need it at this time since my jaw clenching as subsided due to the help from a new prescription that I take called Flexeril, which is a strong muscle relaxer. It works very well for me, along with Advil, and I take natural potent antioxidants like Hawaiian Bioastin, which is effective for managing inflammation, muscle recovery, and acts as a natural sun protector for the skin. One cup of coffee daily, or a Black Tea, White Tea, Green Tea, and Acai Berry for energy and health. Melatonin and Sleepytime Wellness Teas for the evenings. These have made all the positive difference in managing my stress, anxiety, insomnia, and chronic inflammation and pain. Having gingivitis or gum disease means there is inflammation in the gums, and that the immune system is working overtime to combat the bad bacteria. So give your immune system a boost whenever you can. I also take a packet of Emergen-C every morning and evening, this is loaded with vitamin C, it has seven B vitamins, and twenty four nutrients. My favorite is natural tangerine, I mix it with a small amount of water and it tastes great. Do everything that you can to take care of your health. I have new cavities and fillings that are needed, and around the end of this year I can afford to get the work done. I need the more expensive white resin fillings. Never again will I get the pollutant toxic metal fillings that leak mercury. I advise that you do the same. My dentist referred me to a specialist to have an old root canal job redone. The bacteria that has leaked under the gold cap and tooth needs to be cleaned out from under the tooth. Then a new gold cap will be fitted, and because this is the last tooth in the farthest back area of the bottom row, it is not necessary to spend the extra money in having a porcelain cover put over the gold to match my other teeth. I only need that additional work done if it is a tooth that shows when smiling. I hope this time around it will be done correctly and permanently. I am still haunted by the memory of that particular root canal. The farther back in the mouth that they are, the more painful it is going to be. It takes longer, is much more difficult to keep the mouth open wider, and to have Dentist's hands in the back of the mouth, versus working on teeth closer to the front. The exhaustion and pain felt in the jaw is severe, and it is a big deal to just get through it without running out of the office.

7

Various Products and Results

My first problems with this back tooth began when I was coaching gymnastics, I was spotting the students for handstands, and one of the girls threw her legs out the incorrect way clobbering me in the back jaw area by accident. Next visit to the dentist revealed decay and I was in need of a root canal. I remember how extremely difficult it was to hold my mouth that wide and for that long while they worked all the way in the back of my mouth. I had a lot of pain and discomfort, and the doctor gave me a prescription for painkiller pills, I think it was Percocet. Then at the same time I had a broken down car, so a friend of mine was helping me shop around for cars by driving me around town. I had almost two thousand dollars on me for a down payment. Can you believe that when I was high on them pain pills I went lollygagging around a store, and when I had looked at key chains with other stuff in my hand, I dropped one of the key chains in my purse. Turns out I was right in front of a two way window. Security stopped me as soon as I exited the store. I was arrested, and the cops could not believe that I had done that with all the money I had in my purse. I told them I honestly never intended to steal anything, I was high on my prescribed pain pills for the painful procedure I just had done, and I honestly did not recall how it made it into my purse. Minor misdemeanor for me, most embarrassing and I have never taken any kind of prescription painkiller pill since the incident. Now all of these years later, I have to relive that kind of pain again, and with only the help of Advil this time. My current problem is that my dentist feels it would be best to have another more specialized dentist do the procedure, but he does not accept my insurance, and the cost will be more than a thousand. I will need to wait until the end of the year when I can cover the costs. Money is the only thing holding me back. There are many treatments available. If money is of no concern to you, then talk with your hygienist and dental care team and become informed as to what extra treatment options are available at the time that you go in for your teeth and gum maintenance care. There are laser treatments and medications available. The sooner you care for your teeth, the better chance you have of keeping them. I repeat, the sooner you care for your teeth, the better chance you have of keeping them. If I ever repeat myself, it is because repetition equals remembrance. I have been seeing my current hygienist whenever I can afford the copay for cleaning and gum maintenance, every three months is the suggested schedule for me. I can say she is the best hygienist that I have seen yet, and I genuinely really like her. I feel very comfortable being open with her, and I appreciate her knowledge and that she cares to share important tips with me. For as long as I can remember every single hygienist likes to talk story while cleaning my mouth. Maybe that is their way of distracting the patient from discomfort. It works, although occasionally I find myself talking back while nodding, and that is a hard thing to do with a hand and long metal instruments in my mouth. She informed me of the health risks, and that scared me in to further research on the subject, and to learn as much as I could. It has been a real eye opener, and gave me the insight and will power to make changes with my habits and my oral health care routine. I am determined to improve my oral health. It is crucial to have a great dental team helping, and that the office is keeping you on track with appointments. I am not the easiest person to reach by phone, and I have a poor habit of not returning calls right away. My dental office does not give up on me, and I need that. Eventually I will make that appointment and go. After my first visit they gave me a little care package with a toothbrush, a small tube of Colgate Total Fresh Gel, and Reach's Gum Care

Fluoride Woven Floss. I thought that sounded great and could not wait to try them. I loved the toothpaste, but not so much the floss, I felt very disappointed. The woven material floss would sometimes get stuck in my teeth, and I seriously worried that I might pull out a tooth with it. So I went back to using my bag of plastic disposable toothpicks. Now if these plastic picks that so many people use are the only way a person can floss, maybe due to arthritis or such, it is better than nothing. But for me at stage two of this disease it is a shame that I wasted so much time using the plastic ones. A few months later on my second visit to the dental office, I did mention to my hygienist the uncomfortable experience I had with the woven floss. So this time they sent me home with a little round white glide floss in my care package. When I used this floss I was sure that I had just cut my gums and that they were probably bleeding. I looked in the mirror and saw that they were okay, so I pulled another piece through my teeth and gums, and again it felt like they were being cut up. I was done with trying that one, and went back to the plastic picks. With these picks I can only go up and down in between my teeth removing food particles and germs. Research has taught us that not only do we have to focus on cleaning in between the teeth, but also just as importantly under the gum line in the front and the back of our teeth where the bacteria thrives. What I needed was glide floss that does not hurt, and after six months of attempting to incorporate better flossing habits, I discovered the new Oral B Glide Pro-Health Floss. It positively changed my flossing routine, and was heaven to my gums. A couple months later I spotted a new Oral B Clinical Protection Floss, and started using that one. Later on I will tell you why I gave Reach's Gum Care Fluoride Woven Floss another try, and I now use it along with my Oral B Clinical Protection Glide Floss, Reach's Total Care with ridges, and Dr. Tung's Smart Floss, which is my favorite floss. I keep my mouth hydrated with water, since I suffer dry mouth due to meds, and take small sips regularly. I avoid all mouthwashes, only using my toothpaste as a mouthwash, and keep my saliva's enzymes healthy, so that they can keep my mouth moisturized, and fight germs and odors naturally. Having a dry mouth alone can destroy your teeth and gums. I tried Biotene's mouthwash and gum, intended to coat the mouth with enzymes that mimic our saliva. It was recommended to me by another hygienist, and I had watched the commercials for it, so I gave it a try. After a few uses I was able to determine that it left me feeling nauseas, and I stopped using it. I do like the Colgate Total gel because I do not experience any dry mouth after using it. This kind of antibacterial toothpaste with fluoride fights the germs longer. After I brush for the second time, I will then put a dab of toothpaste in my mouth, and then a small amount of warm water. I swish it around my teeth and gums, and swish it from side to side. Spit it out and do not rinse with any water. Making sure to spit a couple of times to get any excess out so as not to swallow any. Last step of my routine will be to rinse the outside of my mouth with cold water and then apply lotion to soothe my sensitive skin. I will have a light burning sensation inside my mouth, but then it quickly subsides. I feel it working in the infected pockets of my gums and I am thinking, die germs, destroy thy enemy. When I began my mission to achieve a healthier mouth, I stopped using gum and candies, and eventually stopped drinking my favorite high sugar juices that I thought I needed for energy at work. I will only drink one hundred percent orange, apple, or pineapple juice, and I always dilute it with water. When I consume something with a lot of sugar or acids, I feel a slight stinging sensation in my gum's pockets. This also happens when I consume anything spicy, so I try to avoid these types of foods.

8

Healthy Approach Foods and Supplements

I decided I was going to try a more natural approach and began using arm and hammer baking soda as a tooth paste. I also mixed baking soda with water, put it in a plastic bottle, and used it as a mouthwash. It felt great, clean, fresh, and without any uncomfortable side effects. I had run out of my Colgate Total gel and prescription fluoride toothpaste at this time, and I was using regular fluoride toothpaste along with the baking soda. By the end of the week the pockets in one area of my upper mouth were enlarged. Pulling away from my teeth, my gum line had receded deeper and I could trace my tongue along it feeling this new hole that spanned across the back of my tooth. I panicked. I immediately went back to using my Colgate Total Gel toothpaste, also using it as my mouthwash, and flossing daily. Soon after that I picked up my prescription fluoride toothpaste. Within two weeks the pocket shrank, and closed up most of the way. My gums slightly adhered back to my teeth. I have a deeper pocket than what had been there previously. If I ever go without flossing or brushing before falling asleep, due to exhaustion or sickness, this pocket will be slightly enlarged by the morning. I can feel the differences with my tongue. The battle is on, and the germ army in my mouth is trying to take over again. I have to brush and floss as much as possible, and keep up to date on my cleanings and gum maintenance. This is going to be a fight for the rest of my life. I have to think of this gum disease as a destructive army that lives in my mouth, and every day I have to fight it. I want to keep my teeth. I want good health. I am making the changes and putting in the effort. I am fighting to keep my teeth and save my life. So should you. Here are some important things to remember and practice in order to keep or obtain a healthy mouth. Always brush and floss every morning and especially every evening before going to bed. Use warm water. Rinse first, brush for two minutes, floss, brush again for two minutes, during which you should clean your brush and swipe it along the top of your mouth, cheeks, and tongue. This process will help keep bad breath odors away much longer during the day, and keep your morning poo breath away. If you are practicing these tips and still suffer from bad breath odor, or halitosis, then consume the purest form of Chlorophyll that you can find, and use it on a daily basis. I use Hawaiian Spirulina because it is also rich in nutrients and chlorophyll. Use toothpicks or wisp brushes to pick out the food between brushing and flossing. Brush with a toothpaste that will treat and prevent gingivitis and fight bio plaque. Use a quality electric toothbrush, or a toothbrush with a gum stimulator. Use a gum stimulator pick. It is a rubber pick that my hygienist gave me on my last visit. I put a tiny bit of my prescription fluoride on the end of it and gently massage it around the exact place of your gum line that connects your teeth and gums. Electric

WaterPiks are helpful in removing plaque as well. I prefer the Oral B Clinical Protection toothbrush with a gum stimulator. Keep a small bottle of dish soap near sink and rub a small dab of it on your toothbrush and rinse before using and after use as well. This will eliminate the transfer of nasty germs going back in to your mouth. Store your toothbrush in a sanitary place, where it can dry, and away from the toilet. A study proved that fecal bacteria is spread through the air when flushing toilets, and was found on peoples toothbrushes. Keep your mouth hydrated, prevent dry mouth by drinking water, sip it and swish it around your mouth periodically. If you smoke, quit smoking, if you chew tobacco, quit now, nicotine will destroy your teeth and gums like a rapid forest fire. Always brush after smoking, and again keep mouth hydrated with water. Strive for a diet that will promote healthy bone and gum tissue. We need calcium for healthy teeth, gums, and bones. Eat low fat dairy products like yogurt that contain probiotics, which are friendly bacteria, that fights off any harmful bacteria. Cut back on foods containing sugar and starches. Eat oatmeal, fortified breakfast cereals, milk, cheese, orange juice, noni fruit, soy and rice drinks. Fatty fish like perch or rainbow trout, salmon or sardines with the bones. Almonds, sesame seeds, chia seeds, flax seed, quinoa, dark green leafy vegetables, broccoli, kale, okra, collards, soy beans, white beans, tofu, molasses, dried fruits like figs, dried herbs, and moderate exposure to the sun are superb sources of calcium. You need vitamin D to help absorb the calcium. It is a lot harder to get enough vitamin D from foods. Aside from a short time spent in the sun to get your body producing vitamin D naturally, eating healthy fats like nuts and avocados, beef liver, fish like mackerel or tuna, oysters, caviar, cod liver oil, coconut oil, olive oil, shitake or button mushrooms. Vitamin D fortified drinks like milk or orange juice, cheese, and egg yolks are high in Vitamin D. So eat healthy with lots of calcium rich foods, take a supplement with a combination of calcium, magnesium, and vitamin D3, is the best. I recommend taking Hawaiian Spirulina because it is rich in nutrients and chlorophyll. I mix a teaspoon of the powder in a glass of water, and I add a bit of natural juice for a better taste. I have read opposite research outcomes on the subject of chlorophyll, and here is what I know from my own personal use. When I do not get enough chlorophyll in my body I stink when I sweat, smelling like the cup of coffee that I drank that morning, which kind of reminds me of the smell of cat pee. Eewww I know. Chlorophyll makes my sweat odors smell sweet. That is nice. Living on an Island that has an active volcano, I suffer from the VOG, which is volcanic fog. I have noticed that the more VOG in the air, the more intense my fatigue and body aches feel. I consume Hawaiian Spirulina daily, it puts oxygen in my blood, I smell good, I have more energy, and I notice my breath is fresher. It counteracts the acids in my stomach, decreasing any chance of heartburn. Super good stuff! Get enough sleep and try to avoid stress. Do not kiss anyone with an unhealthy mouth. Do not kiss a healthy mouth if your mouth is unhealthy. I am talking about the intimate way that adults like to kiss, open mouthed, and they trade a lot of saliva between them. The beloved French kiss. Do not share glasses or utensils. A person could unknowingly give it to their spouse or children. The different types of bacteria can be transferred through the saliva. Give up eating and drinking any sugar, or as much as possible. Switch drinking habits from soda and sugar juices to water. Add cucumber or lemon to your water to satisfy your cravings and thirst. The bonus benefit of adding cucumber to your water is its effect in helping you feel calm for up to four hours after consuming. Do not chew gum or eat candy. Choose something that you will like, and that is healthy to take its place. Fruits are no longer the recommended snack for in between meals because of the high acidity and sugar which erode teeth. Dried fruits will stick to the teeth allowing the sugar to settle in. It has been revealed that apples can be as bad as sweets and fizzy drinks. Fruits sugar content has risen by as much as fifty percent over the last decade, with so much more sweeter varieties available. Fruits should be consumed with meals. Fruit juices should be diluted before drinking them. Always rinse your mouth out with warm water right after eating meals, since this will also help to prevent brushing away any enamel that is softened from the acids in your foods. Carry your toothpaste, toothbrush, and floss with you. Use a tiny dab of toothpaste in your mouth for a quick fresh breath fix. If my teeth and gums were healthy, I would most likely be using the new Tom's Natural Toothpaste with Fluoride. It has a smaller amount of fluoride as regular toothpaste, and contains xylitol, which is a natural sweetener that may reduce the risk of tooth decay. I bought a bottle of xylitol for twenty five dollars from my dental office on my last visit. I will put two pieces in my mouth, up to three times a day, and let it dissolve into my saliva and coat my teeth. It tastes great. I can only hope that it will help. My son uses Tom's toothpaste now, and he really likes the way it tastes. It is too late for me to use any natural toothpaste, being at stage two of periodontal gum disease, it would do me more harm than good to stop using fluoride. The damage I have is irreversible, and all I can do is manage it, trying my best to prevent progression. I need to use fluorides. Have a great hygienist and dentist, see them regularly for exams, cleanings, and gum maintenance. There is some good news, teeth and bones are able to heal themselves in a process of remineralization. The important factors are having enough minerals and A, D, E, and K vitamins in the diet. How bio-available these nutrients are and how well the body is absorbing them, is mostly influenced by the presence of phytic acid in the diet. Higher rates of tooth decay, mineral deficiencies and osteoporosis were found in people who eat large amounts of phytic acid in the form of nuts, seeds, grains, and legumes. So eat them in moderation. Also it is good to know that it is healthy to eat a low fat diet. We need to consume healthy fats, like avocados. Doctors hypothesized that these factors control the body's ability to reverse cavities and oral health problems, and that if you could enhance these factors, you could prevent further damage and reverse any present damage.

9
Proper Oral Care for Children

Research has proven that children and adults who do not receive proper dental care, and have problems or pain persisting in their mouths, are unable to focus in their academics and work life. This leads to social and economic failure. Proper care begins before a child's teeth even come in. Avoid BBTD, baby bottle tooth decay, by not giving them a crib bottle. Bottles should only been given at feedings, separate the last bottle given of the evening from bedtime, and going in to the crib. Do not substitute with a pacifier, toy, object, or being held. If you must give them a bottle, then fill it with water only. This is not as exciting and will ultimately help them get off the bottle and to using cups. Weaning them from the bottle to cups can sometimes take up to three months. Before babies teeth come in, an adult should wipe the gums with a clean damp gauze or washcloth that is free of laundry soap or chemicals and perfumes from dryer sheets. Rinse and ring out the cloth under hot water several times before using it. Make sure to open up the cloth to let the steam out and cool before placing in the child's mouth. Once the teeth have come in, brush them twice a day. Use a soft toothbrush with polished nylon bristles. Wet the toothbrush in hot water for a few seconds to make the bristles clean and soft, use cool water before putting inside a child's mouth. Start using fluoridated toothpaste when the child is two years old. Use only a tiny dab of toothpaste, like the size of a child's pinky fingernail. Young children often swallow toothpaste when brushing rather than spitting it out. This can sometimes lead to fluorosis and cosmetic problems in the permanent teeth. As soon as two teeth touch each other, floss between them once a day with regular floss or plastic floss picks. If your child does not drink water that is fluoridated, talk to your doctor or dentist about needing fluoride treatments or supplements. When a child is ready to start brushing on their own, give them the brush and teach them the proper way. Afterward you should brush your child's teeth for a second time. Most children are not adequate enough to brush their teeth well until they are eight years old. Sealants can be placed on teeth of children who are at high risk for cavities. These are plastic coverings that are placed over the grooves of teeth to protect them from decay. One in seven grade school age children in my state of Hawaii suffer from a toothache. These children lack the ability to focus their attention on their schoolwork, and they miss numerous school days. I have learned that Hawaii has the lowest level of fluoride in the water system. I checked with my community of Waikoloa's water system to see if they add fluoride to my water, and learned that they do not. This is a good thing for me because I use prescription fluoride toothpaste daily, and I do not want to overexpose myself to any medicinal toxic chemical. I also check the labels of bottled water that I buy, some may contain fluoride, and I do not need any extra in my water. I have come to my own conclusion and belief that controlled use of fluoride is highly important. If a child or adult is drinking fluoridated water, then they should limit other uses of fluoride. If the water they drink does not contain it, it would be beneficial to use toothpastes, mouth rinses, and tablets with fluoride.

10
Caution Fluoride Facts

Fluoride compounds are salts that form when the element, fluorine, combines with minerals in soil or rocks. It is found naturally in soil, water, foods, and minerals. Sodium fluoride is a hazardous by product made from the waste streams of metal, aluminum, and nuclear factories, and the phosphate fertilizer industry. These waste fluorides might be laced with impurities such as arsenic, lead, chromium, and other proven carcinogens. This is why there is so much controversial dispute about it. Many communities add sodium fluoride to their drinking water to promote dental health. There is some concern for caution of fluorides health effects. Synthesized fluorides are not as good has the natural occurring kind. Over exposure to plethoric consumption of fluoride during a lifetime may lead to escalated plausibility of bone fractures in adults, and may result in effects on bone leading to pain and tenderness. Children under eight years of age whom are exposed to excessive amounts of fluoride have an elevated chance of developing pits in the tooth enamel, along with a realm of cosmetic effects to teeth. In India an estimated sixty million people have been poisoned by well water contaminated by excessive fluoride, which is dissolved from the granite rocks. The effects are particularly evident in the bone deformations of children. Similar or larger problems are anticipated in other countries including China,

Uzbekistan, and Ethiopia. Consumption of fluoride at levels beyond those used in fluoridated water for a long period of time causes skeletal fluorosis. In some areas, particularly the Asian subcontinent, skeletal fluorosis is endemic. It is known to cause irritable bowel symptoms and joint pain. Early stages are not clinically obvious, and may be misdiagnosed as rheumatoid arthritis or ankylosing spondylitis. Which is a chronic inflammatory disease of the axial skeleton with variable involvement of peripheral joints, and it mainly affects joints in the spine and the sacroiliac joint in the pelvis, and can cause eventual fusion of the spine. I have read shocking historical documentation that implies Hitler and the German Nazi's adopting a plan to control the population in any given area through mass medication of drinking water supplies. Using this method they could control the population in whole areas, produce sterility in women, and make people more docile. Repeated doses of infinitesimal amounts of fluoride will in time reduce an individual's power to resist domination, by slowly poisoning and narcotizing a certain area of the brain, making him submissive to the will of those who wish to govern him. Equivalent to that of an easy light lobotomy. Now that sounds like some scary stuff. It raises that caution flag, but we also have to determine the health needs of our mouth. The more severe the teeth and gum problems are, the more at risk for serious health problems, organ damage, heart attack and stroke. These problems can kill, and they are very difficult to overcome. If you feel that you need to use an extra strength fluoride like I do, then use it wisely, and be mindful of overexposure. Do not ingest it, and always expectorate it from your mouth and lungs.

11
Promote or Prevention

Prevention is the key. From the time I started writing this book, I have learned that many people I know are seeking out dental services. One day I took my son to our dentist for his exam and cleaning, and while I was there I saw an associate from work. He said he is having some problems with his teeth, I asked if he flosses, and he replied no. I told him that he is going to need to start now or his problems are only going to get worse, that the only way to hopefully reverse whatever stage his teeth problems are in, is by daily brushing and flossing. And to start using prescription fluoride, antibacterial, and antigingivitis toothpaste. I have several friends that have not been seeing a dentist regularly. They brush daily, and floss only sometimes. Their gums bleed when they floss. Some friends said they are starting to get the deep pockets around their teeth and gums. They feel the irritation and discomfort from the inflammation. One friend whom is without any dental insurance is making financial sacrifices in order to pay for her dental care with cash. Another friend without any dental coverage applied and signed herself up on a list of people who will receive dental services at majorly discounted prices. Other friends say that they are not having any current problems with their teeth. They brush day and night, and do not floss. They said that when they do floss their gums will bleed. That tells me that they have gingivitis or some worse stage of gum disease. Just because they are not experiencing any discomfort, does not mean that they can assume that they have a healthy mouth. Healthy gums do not bleed when brushing and flossing. They would normally be quite strong, and there should be no discomfort. The normal color for gums is described as coral pink. Unhealthy gums will have an ashen look, greyish white, or red. My gums are a light pink, but I am seeing a red line that traces right along my gum line and my teeth. It has become more noticeable to me since I allowed my gum disease to have its way, and my condition has slightly worsened.

12
Unforeseeable Changes

While working on this book, and making an effort to improve the health of my teeth and gums, my life went spinning out of control and seemed to perpetuate a lot more stress. My unsympathetic landlord forced us to evacuate with our pets for two days while he tent fumigated our home with a gas that kills termites and everything. Then soon after that, the day before Thanksgiving, two dogs that were running around loose in our neighborhood, spotted my cat Blackie sleeping in the sun by our front door, and they attacked and killed her. I was hurt badly during the horrific ordeal, needing an emergency doctor's visit to treat my wounds and they gave me a tetanus shot. My son came home from work and mopped and cleaned up the bloody mess. My son was such a great help to me while I was healing. He did everything around the house for two weeks. After two weeks I was finally feeling better, and for Christmas my greedy landlord served us a certified letter to tell us he would not be renewing our lease. He wanted to renovate and charge more money. We had two months to find a new home and move. This was at the worst time of year. I was super busy at work during the Holiday season, and hardly any rentals were available, especially ones that would allow dogs and cats. I felt like a poker player, holding out for the home that we wanted, and the risk being that we could end up homeless. Thank god we got the house that we wanted, and moved into a more expensive larger home that is closer to my work. Now with all that I just shared with you, I am sure you can understand how and why my teeth and gums suffered a setback. Not only from the stress that my immune system has had to work overtime to combat, but also because I stopped flossing and was only brushing. I noticed I was getting headaches that were a direct result from my gums inflammation. Anytime there is food debris left in between my teeth for any length of time, I get an associated headache. When I floss and brush, my gums feel better, and so does my head. As soon as I settled into our new home, I got back on track with my oral health care regimen of brushing and flossing. My headaches subsided, and I made an appointment for my teeth and gum maintenance cleaning. I decided not to do any x-rays at this time, because why would I want to expose myself to radiation for nothing. I know what all of my current problems are, and I do not have the funds available to do any needed procedures right now. I will do exams later when I have the money to proceed with fixing anything more.

13
Best Products, Techniques, and Procedures

They have a new tool that can measure the depth of the pockets of each tooth. They slide it over each tooth and it will tell them if it is a one, two, three, four or five. This time around I had more fours and a few fives. Not good, and I needed to pay an extra hundred dollars for an antibiotic powder to be put in between two of my back teeth. The pocket is so deep that flossing alone will never get it to close. So they put in this powder, and I was not allowed to floss that area for two weeks. I was encouraged to come back for a deep cleaning, where they lift up the gum line to remove more plaque. I also still need fillings and to have a new root canal done. I do not have the money. It has been a struggle to get back into routine of flossing before bedtime. It has been much harder to start flossing before leaving for work. I am coming to realize once again, that if I do not do this every day and night, I will eventually lose my teeth. Possibly my life from the potential damage that the bacteria may cause to my organs. Not having the money to pay for treatments that I need means brushing, flossing, and using gum stimulators every morning and evening are going to be my best weapons. I am dedicated to preventing any further progression. I will seek out more help as soon as I can afford the necessary treatments. It hurts a little bit like when I first started flossing before, but each day becomes less irritating, and my gums are getting stronger, and feeling better. I believe that my commitment to consistency will bring positive results. I cannot stop or fall behind ever again. I know how crucial it is to not let my guard down by being lazy with my routine. No matter what life may throw my way, and it throws me some real curve balls. You know the kind, the real doozies that take time to recover from. I just had another appointment with my hygienist for a regular cleaning while I wrap up the end of this book. That was all that I can afford at this time. I had brushed and flossed with my Oral B Clinical Protection Glide Floss the night before, the only floss I had at the time, and I did not eat in the morning before my appointment. I brushed my teeth quickly before making the hour long drive to Kailua Kona town. My hygienist gave me a mirror to hold to watch as she flossed my teeth with Reach's Gum Care Fluoride Woven Floss. I could not believe how much food and plaque she cleaned out from between my teeth. I thought they were clean, I could not have been more wrong. My comfortable glide floss is not removing all of the debris. Those tiny particles do not stick to the smooth floss. So now I use the Oral B Clinical Protection Floss as a way to get the antibacterial medicine up and under the gum line, sliding it back and forth. To remove more plaque from between my teeth I use Reach's Gum Care with Fluoride Woven Floss, it takes a bit of getting used to, it can hurt my sometimes sore fingers, and on occasion it will get stuck in between the teeth and that is annoying, or if I pull it out too hard and catch it on a tooth. To eliminate this problem I have learned to hold it very tight and to use a new spot for every tooth. I also use Reach's Total Care Floss, with ridges, and Dr. Tung's Smart Floss is my best choice. These flosses stretch, are very comfortable to use, and catch a lot more debris. My hygienist gave me two red tablets to help improve brushing and flossing in areas that I am missing. All you do is chew them up, and look in the mirror to see if there are any red spots. Those red spots are the places where there is still plaque, then focus better on cleaning in those places. TheraMints Xylitol tablets are available as well, if you want to try them for around twenty five dollars a bottle. All I know is I really enjoy the naturally sweet little tablets, and even better is thinking that they may reduce tooth decay. My hygienist convinced me that I need to do my oral cleanings in front of a mirror. She told me that one day she had flossed without looking in the mirror, and she had missed two different places. No matter how experienced you are, it does make a difference to use a mirror. Occasionally I add one last step to my brush, floss, and brush routine. I will swallow one tablespoon of organic unrefined coconut oil for my overall health, then I put one tablespoon of coconut oil in my mouth, and I brush it all around my mouth, and spit out the excess. This is to aid in the cleansing and healing process of my entire mouth. It feels great, just try it. Opt for a dental team that uses the cool new laser technology I mentioned before, called the DIAGNOdent. This small laser instrument scans the teeth with harmless laser light searching for decay. Locating hidden decay before it destroys tooth structure, from the inside out, is a major goal for modern dentistry. While the widespread use of fluoride supplements in dental materials, toothpastes, and drinking water have made tooth surfaces harder and more resistant to decay. The disease process can start through microscopic defects in the hard surface enamel and can readily spread into the softer tooth structure beneath the surface. This unique instrument provides instant feedback on the health of the tooth. It's a pen like probe that glides over the tooth surface. A number scale and an alarm signal the operator when there are signs of hidden decay. It is safe and pain free. We learned I have a new cavity trying to form on the top right side of my mouth. She measured the depth of my pockets around my teeth. The number scale starts with one and went up to five. It sounded a lot like this when she moved the instrument from tooth to tooth. Two, two, three, three, three, four, four, and I had a five in the same place as I did from my prior visit. That time I paid extra to have an antibacterial powder inserted. This time my funds are limited and I had to pass on any extra treatment. My hygienist informed me that if this five progresses into a measured depth of a six, there will be no hope of it ever closing from just flossing alone. Special procedures will be needed to help the health of those teeth. The great news is that there are many things available at different cost levels to help fight gingivitis and gum disease. It is important to remember that if you just have gingivitis, you can rid yourself of it through proper oral care and treatments. Once you allow it to progress to any stage of gum disease, it is incurable, and you can only keep it from further progression through proper oral care and treatments. The first stage is gingivitis, the second stage is periodontitis, the third stage is advanced periodontitis, and the fourth stage is severely advanced periodontitis, usually resulting in loss of teeth. That is why the fight is on to prevent further progression. To share some other new things that I learned on my last visit, let me tell you about Opalescence. It is a new powerful, effective, and safer bleaching procedure to whiten your teeth. Opalescence toothpaste is available to maintain your smile. There is a ceramic restoration procedure called CEREC. If you want highly aesthetic, tooth colored filings created and placed in one single visit, bonded directly to your tooth. Enduring only one painful visit sounds super to me, and I am sure that you would agree. So ask your dental professional team more about these new procedures, if that is something of interest to you. We discussed the reality of my finances and that all of my money goes to my living expenses. This means it is a crucial time for me to increase my focus on my oral health care. Dental professionals recommend Philips Sonicare electric toothbrushes, so I bought a two pack for my son and I, and he loves his, but me not so much. The buzzing going on in my mouth, is felt all in my head, and my head is usually sore and tired whenever brushing. So I use the best manual Oral B Clinical Protection Toothbrush that I can find with a gum stimulator. I feel like my tongue gets much cleaner when I use the bristles of my toothbrush rather than a tongue scraper. Do this in the shower and let the water run down the tongue at the same time you are brushing it. This will help reduce any gagging, and also leaves your tongue very clean and fresh. Follow my brushing and flossing system. Wash it with dish soap daily, and replace it every two to three months.

14
Review Important Reminders

Never go to sleep with poo in the mouth. Use Reach's Gum Care Fluoride Woven Floss, Reach's Total Care Floss with ridges, its stretchy and comfortable in the mouth and fingers, and Dr. Tung's Smart Floss is natural, stretchy, comfortable, and expands in between the teeth. It is my favorite floss. I have a cool new trick that I do with Mr. Tung's Floss, I rub a dab of toothpaste in between my fingers, and then I rub my fingers all along my string of floss before using it. It is very effective, I can feel it working, and the spaces in between my teeth are fresher, while it is killing the germs in there. Oral B Clinical Protection Floss is good for getting the antibacterial medicine under the gum line too. These are the best flossing products to remove more plaque between the teeth and gums, than any other floss that I have tried. I like to carry with me tiny antibacterial wisp brushes for in between my teeth. They come in sizes for tight, medium, or wide teeth. I use the tight wisp brush since my teeth are close together, and I carry them with me. Remember to brush, floss, and brush again every morning and night. Invest in a more costly type of Oral B toothbrush with a Gum Stimulator. Use a Gum Stimulator Pick with a bit of fluoride on the end, and glide around your gum line. Use a prescription, if needed, or regular fluoride toothpaste. Use warm water if possible. Do use a mirror. Preferably over a sink. Use pure unprocessed coconut oil to aid in the cleansing and healing of your entire mouth. Take a teaspoon of it daily for optimal health, and to control the growth of yeast in the mouth and body. Do not eat or drink for thirty minutes after cleaning teeth, and only have water if it is at bedtime. Stay on schedule with visits to the hygienist for cleanings and gum maintenance every three months. Do not over fluorinate by exposing yourself to too much fluoride. Eat and drink healthy foods that will promote a healthy mouth. Strive for calcium and Vitamin D rich foods and supplements. Stay away from acidic drinks and foods that will erode the enamel. Eat yogurt with probiotics, or take a probiotic supplement to boost your immune system. Do not chew gum or eat candy. If you must chew gum, look for Peelu Gum, sweetened with xylitol. It is a great new product that I buy sometimes, since it is made with fibers of the Peelu tree, which is said to brighten teeth naturally. My favorite is citrus breeze with vitamin C, or vanilla mint. The flavor runs out fast, but I keep it in my mouth for a while to clean my teeth. TheraMints with xylitol in a tasty fruit or mint flavor may help fight tooth decay. I like to keep my breath fresh, and say no to poo mouth. And so should you. Keep hydrated with water. I buy most of my supplements at Costco for the excellent savings, but they are available at most drug stores, and online. Hawaiian Spirulina has pure chlorophyll, and nutrients to ensure fresh breath, and good health. Hawaiian Bioastin, it is a super potent natural antioxidant, and helps with managing inflammation in the whole body, and provides your skin with a natural sun protector. I have started taking MegaRed Omega-3 Krill Oil. This supports heart and joint health, as well as brain function, better thinking, and sleeping. Without fishy after taste, or smell, and no burps. Manage your stress, and make getting enough sleep a priority. I just got back from yet another visit with my hygienist, and as always, a much needed cleaning. She told me there is an improvement in the health of my gums, more on the top, than the bottom, but still an improvement. I heard more twos and threes, and less fours and fives. This is good. We hope for more progressive results on the next visit. My gums are responding quickly again to flossing. Becoming stronger, healthier, and feeling better each day. My headaches have subsided. I constantly remind myself that if I ever stop flossing my gums, they will just as quickly deteriorate again. This is going to be a lifetime battle for me. Writing this book and sharing the knowledge that I have gained through my experience and diligent research, has helped me tremendously. In the future I will write a follow up and share the status of my oral health. I would like to thank you for taking the time to read my first book, and allowing me to entertain you with parts of my life, and how it correlates to my struggle with gum disease. Most importantly, I hope to have helped you gain knowledge and motivation to ensure your own optimal oral health care, and overall good health. Now go brush and floss every day, and keep those germs away. Defend yourself against this deadly disease.

Author's Note

I have other writing project ideas to embark on, such as a review on how I improved my ear tinnitus, and reduced my suffering. The juicy details of living for nine months without power and water half of the time on the Caribbean Island of Roatan, Honduras. I plan to create a children's story, and a book about cats. I also have other visions in mind. I will update any future work in progress on my website, and I wish for everyone to read as soon as anything new comes out.

Visit my website to order cool shirts, hats, and hoodies, with more stuff soon to come. My goal is to offer comfort wear, with cute, and classy designs. With options to choose small, or large designs, printed on the front, or back, and what item you want to wear it on. Many designs I create are inspired by my love for the Hawaiian Islands.

morgansbooksshirtsandmore.com

Visit my animal charity website to view pictures of cats that I care for, with much needed help, from my terrific son. Any donation would be greatly appreciated by us, especially the cats. We aim to help other kinds of animals in the future.

helphomelessanimalsinhawaii.org

3

Super Delicious Avocado Custard

Total time: 1 hr

Servings: 4

Ingredients:

- ☐ 4 large eggs

- ☐ 2 medium avocados, mashed

- ☐ ½ cup coconut milk

- ☐ 1/3 cup heavy cream

- ☐ 1/3 cup erythritol

- ☐ 1/3 cup almond butter

- ☐ 1 tsp vanilla extract

- ☐ 1 tsp liquid stevia

Directions:

Preheat the oven at 325 degrees.

Put all the ingredients in a mixing bowl and whisk them lightly.

Now, fill a baking pan with an inch of water and then put 4 ramekins filled with the custard mixture in the water.

Bake for 40 minutes and make sure that the custard is properly set.

Cool down to room temperature and then keep in the fridge to chill before serving.

Nutrition per Serving

Protein: 6.2g

Fat: 26.2g

Carbohydrate: 2.5g Net

Avocado Delight Ice Cream

Total time: 7 hrs

Serving: 4

Ingredients:

- 1/3 cup erythritol
- 1 cup heavy cream
- 3 large egg yolks
- ½ tsp vanilla extract
- 1 tsp vodka
- 1/8 tsp xanthan gum
- 1 large avocado, mashed

Directions:

Heat up the heavy cream over low flame and then add the erythritol in it. Do not boil but just simmer so that the erythritol is completely dissolved.

Use an immersion blender to beat the egg yolks and then temper the eggs with a few tablespoons of hot cream. Remember to beat constantly.

Now, add the vodka followed by xanthan gum and then place the entire mixture into the ice cream maker and run the device as directed by the manufacturer. Once the cream is chilled add the mashed avocados and let the ice cream chill for 6 more hours.

Serve chilled.

Nutrition per Serving

Protein: 2.3g

Fat: 16.9g

Carbohydrate: 2.3g Net

Utterly-Butterly Avocado Ice Cream

Total time: 1 hr

Servings: 4

Ingredients:

- ¼ cup heavy cream

- 5 tbsp butter

- 1½ cup coconut milk

- 1 large avocado, mashed

- ¼ cup crushed pecans

- ¼ tsp xanthan gum

- 25 drops of liquid stevia

Directions:

Melt the butter over low heat till it turns to amber color. Now add the heavy cream, pecans and stevia and blend with a hand blender to make a smooth paste.

Put coconut milk in a bowl and blend it with the xanthan gum. Now, blend the coconut milk mixture with the butter mixture.

Pour the entire mixture into the ice cream maker and run the device according to the instruction provided by the manufacturer.

Serve chilled by garnishing with some chopped avocados.

Nutrition per Serving

Protein: 0.7g

Fat: 35.3g

Carbohydrate: 1.3g Net

Chocolate & Avocado Double Delight Ice Cream

Total time: 1 hr

Servings: 6

Ingredients:

☐ 1 cup coconut milk

☐ ½ cup heavy cream

☐ 25 drops of liquid stevia

☐ 2 tsp vanilla extract

☐ ½ cup powdered erythritol

☐ 2 ripe avocados

☐ ½ cup cocoa powder

☐ 6 squares of unsweetened chocolate

Directions:

Scoop out the avocado flesh in a bowl and then add coconut milk along with vanilla extract. Use an immersion blender to make a creamy mixture.

Now, add the powdered erythritol along with the liquid stevia and cocoa powder to the mixture of the avocado. Finally add the chocolate pieces into the mixture and distribute them evenly with a spoon. Keep the mixture in the fridge for 12 hours.

Take it out from the fridge and then run it in ice cream machine to make the ice cream.

Nutrition per Serving

Protein: 3g

Fat: 22.7g

Carbohydrate: 3.7g Net

Lemon & Avocado Cake

Total time: 50 mins

Servings: 2

Ingredients:

- [ ] 2 tbsp coconut flour

- [ ] 1 cup almond flour

- [ ] 5 large eggs, separated into whites and yolks

- [ ] 1 tsp baking powder

- [ ] 2 tbsp avocado extract

- [ ] 1 medium avocado, mashed

- [ ] 1 small avocado, diced

- [ ] ¼ tsp liquid stevia

- [ ] ¼ cup erythritol

- [ ] Juice of 1 lime

- [ ] 2 tbsp salted butter

- [ ] ¼ cup cream cheese

- [ ] Zest of 1 lime

Directions:

Keep the oven ready by preheating at 325 degrees.

Mix all the dry ingredients thoroughly and keep aside. Beat the egg yolks in a small bowl till it becomes pale yellow in color.

Add liquid stevia, erythritol, avocado extract, cream cheese and butter to the yolk and remember to beat continuously. Now, add the lime juice (reserve 2 tsp lime juice for later use), mashed avocado and lime zest and beat hard to make the paste smooth.

Add the dry ingredient mixture and blend thoroughly with an immersion blender to make smooth paste.

Beat the egg whites with 2 tsp of lime juice till they form stiff peaks and then fold it to the main mixture. Pour this batter in the loaf pan and top with diced avocados.

Bake for 40 minutes and then allow cooling down.

Slice the cake and serve.

Nutrition per Serving

Protein: 6.4g

Fat: 12.4g

Carbohydrate: 3g Net

Majestic Avocado Sorbet

Total time: 30 mins

Servings: 4

Ingredients:

- ☐ 2 medium sized hash avocado
- ☐ ¼ tsp liquid stevia
- ☐ ¼ cup powdered erythritol
- ☐ 1 cup coconut milk
- ☐ Zest of 2 medium limes
- ☐ Juice of 2 medium limes
- ☐ ½ cup chopped cilantro

Directions:

Cut the avocados into very thin slices along the length and keep them on a foil. Spread lime juice over the avocado slices and keep them in the fridge for at least 3 hours.

Blend erythritol with the zest of 2 limes and coconut milk and bring the mixture to boil over medium heat and let it reduce by 25 %.

Pour in a container and keep in the fridge so that it becomes thick. Put the sliced avocados in food processor and then cover it with chopped cilantro along with the remaining lime juice.

Process them till you have a chunky texture and then add the mixture of coconut milk. Grind the entire mixture till the desired consistency is achieved.

Keep in the fridge for few more hours and serve chilled.

Nutrition per Serving

Protein: 2g

Fat: 16g

Carbohydrate: 3.5g Net

Almond & Avocado Blast

Total time: 20 mins

Servings: 14

Ingredients:

- [ ] 4 tbsp erythritol
- [ ] 2 tbsp butter
- [ ] ¼ tsp liquid stevia
- [ ] ¼ cup heavy cream
- [ ] 1 tbsp + 1 tsp coconut oil
- [ ] ½ cup almonds, toasted
- [ ] 1½ tsp avocado extract
- [ ] ¼ cup chia seeds

- ☐ 2 large avocados, mashed

- ☐ 2 tbsp coconut flour

- ☐ ½ coconut cream

Directions:

Grind the almonds in a food processor till a mealy texture is attained. Add 1 teaspoon of coconut oil with the almonds and 2 tablespoon of erythritol and continue running the food processor to make the almond butter.

Heat the butter in a pan till it turns brown in color and then add the heavy cream along with erythritol, stevia and avocado extract. Keep stirring the mixture continuously and check it is bubbling.

As the almond butter is being incorporated, grind the chia seeds and toast them. Mix all of them in the almond butter mixture along with coconut cream, mashed avocados, coconut oil and coconut flour and spread it in a square dish.

Keep in fridge for at least one hour and then chop into smaller squares before serving.

Nutrition per Serving

Protein: 2.4g

Fat: 11.1g

Carbohydrate: 1.4g Net

Spicy Avocado Fritters with Avocado Glaze

Total time: 15 mins

Servings: 12

Ingredients for spicy fritters:

☐ 1 large egg

☐ 1 tsp baking powder

☐ 3 tbsp erythritol

☐ ½ cup almond flour

☐ ½ tsp cinnamon

☐ ½ tsp xanthan gum

☐ ½ tsp vanilla

☐ 2 cups olive oil (for frying)

☐ Zest of ½ lemon

☐ 1 large semi-ripe avocado, cut into very small pieces

Ingredients for lemon glaze:

☐ 3 tbsp powdered erythritol

☐ 1 tsp avocado extract

☐ ½ tsp lemon juice

Directions:

Mix all the dry ingredients thoroughly and then add the egg to make sticky dough for the fritters. Add the avocado pieces towards the end.

Heat the olive oil in a pan and begin to fry the small balls made from the dough.

Fry 4 balls in each batch and then rest them on paper towels to get rid of the excess oil.

Mix the lemon juice, avocado extract and erythritol in a small bowl to make a smooth icing and then dip the fritter balls to coat them evenly.

Nutrition per Serving

Protein: 1.7g

Fat: 4.6g

Carbohydrate: 0.7g Net

Delicious Cheesy Avocado Tarts

Total time: 1 hr

Servings: 10

Ingredients for making the crust:

- ☐ 2 large eggs

- ☐ ¾ cup coconut flour

- ☐ 8 tbsp salted butter

- ☐ 2 tbsp granulated splenda

Ingredients for avocado cheesecake filling:

- ☐ 3 large eggs

- ☐ 6 oz cream cheese

- ☐ ¾ granulated splenda

- ☐ 1¼ cup avocado flesh

- ☐ 1 tsp Allspice

- ☐ 1 tsp cinnamon

- ☐ 1 tsp vanilla extract

- ☐ ½ tsp ground ginger

Directions:

Blend the butter, eggs and splenda in a bowl to make a smooth liquid and then add the coconut flour to make the dough. Keep the dough in a saran wrap and store in fridge for half an hour so that the dough can set well. Now, take the dough out and mold it in cupcake tins. Bake them in the oven for 6 minutes at 350 degrees, making sure the sides turn golden brown and then keep them aside.

Now, to make the cheesy avocado filling, keep the cream cheese and eggs in a mixing bowl and beat to make it creamier. Use another bowl to mix the splenda, Allspice, cinnamon and ground ginger. In the meantime, add the avocado flesh to the cream cheese and beat them thoroughly and then add the spice mixture to it.

Take the prepared tart crusts and use a spoon to fill them up with the cheesy avocado filling. Allow cooling by keeping them in the fridge and then take out the cakes from the molds to serve.

Nutrition per Serving

Protein: 4.7g

Fat: 16.7g

Carbohydrate: 3.3g Net

Creamy Raspberry & Avocado Popsicles

Total time: 2 hr 5 mins

Servings: 6

Ingredients:

- 1 cup avocado flesh

- 100 g raspberries

- 1 cup coconut milk

- ½ tsp Gaur gum

- ¼ cup sour cream

- ¼ cup heavy cream

- ¼ cup coconut oil

- 20 drops of liquid stevia

Directions:

Put all the ingredients in a large mixing bowl and use a hand blender to make the smooth paste. Use a strainer to remove the seeds of raspberries.

Pour the mixture into Popsicle molds and keep in fridge for at least 2 hours.

Serve chilled.

Nutrition per Serving

Protein: 0.5g

Fat: 16g

Carbohydrate: 2g Net

Super Creamy Avocado Fat Bombs

Total time: 2 hr 5 mins

Servings: 10

Ingredients:

- ☐ 6 oz cream cheese

- ☐ ½ cup coconut oil

- ☐ ½ heavy whipping cream

- ☐ 10 drops of liquid stevia

- ☐ 1 cup mashed avocado

Directions:

Put all the ingredients in a bowl and use an immersion blender to make a smooth paste.

Spread this paste in a silicone tray and keep in fridge for at least 2 hours.

Take out the tray and roll up the mixture to form balls and serve cold.

Nutrition per Serving

Protein: 0.8g

Fat: 20g

Carbohydrate: 0.7g Net

Pudding with Mixture of Mint & Avocado

Total time: 20 mins

Servings: 1

Ingredients:

- ¼ cup coconut milk
- ¼ cup chia seeds
- ½ cup almond milk
- 2 tbsp fresh mint leaves
- 10 drops of stevia extract
- 1 tbsp erythritol
- ¼ cup mashed avocado
- Whipped cream

Directions:

Put the mint leaves along with coconut milk, avocado flesh, and almond milk in blender. Pulse the device to make a smooth paste.

Now, mix the chia seeds with this mixture and then add the erythritol and then add the stevia.

Let the mixture sit for 10 minutes and then keep it in the fridge for overnight before serving the pudding. Serve by topping with whipped cream and some chopped avocado.

Nutrition per Serving

Protein: 9.2g

Fat: 28.8g

Carbohydrate: 6.8g Net

Avocado & Rhubarb Fantasy

Total time: 1 hr

Servings: 12

Ingredients for making the fruit layer:

☐   2 cups of rhubarb

☐   3 large avocados, sliced

☐   ½ tsp cinnamon

☐   2 tbsp ground chia seeds

☐   ¼ cup erythritol

☐   20 drops of stevia

Ingredients for making the crumble:

☐   ½ cup whole almonds

☐   1 cup ground almonds

☐   ¼ cup shredded coconut

☐   ¼ cup whey protein powder

☐   15 drops stevia

☐   ¼ cup erythritol

☐   ¼ cup pecans

☐   ½ cup almond flour

- □   ½ tsp cinnamon

- □   Extract of 1 vanilla bean

- □   1 large egg white

- □   2 tbsp butter

- □   ¼ tsp salt

Directions:

Keep the oven ready by preheating it at 40 degrees.

Keep the avocado slices and rhubarb in a baking dish and add the cinnamon, stevia and erythritol and bake for 30 minutes. Then keep them aside by mixing the ground chia seeds. Bring down the oven temperature to 300 degrees.

Make the crumble by mixing all the ingredients thoroughly. Place them on the baking tray and cook for 20 minutes, making sure that the batter is evenly distributes in the tray. Remove from oven and allow cooling before serving.

Nutrition per Serving

Protein: 4.9g

Fat: 14.6g

Carbohydrate: 3.8g Net

Easy keto Ice Cream with Ripe Avocado

Total time: 1 hr

Servings: 8

Ingredients:

- ½ cup butter

- ½ cup coconut oil

- 4 large egg yolks

- 2 large eggs

- 30 drops of stevia

- ¼ cup erythritol

- 2 large avocado, mashed

- 1 tsp avocado extract

- 1 cup coconut milk

Directions:

Blend butter, coconut oil, avocado extract, mashed avocado, erythritol and stevia and then add the egg yolks slowly with this mixture. Put them in food processor and pulse to make a smooth paste.

Pour in the coconut milk and keep pulsing.

Put the entire mixture into the ice cream maker and process as directed by the manufacturer. It will take about an hour.

Serve chilled by garnishing with avocado slices.

Nutrition per Serving

Protein: 3.6g

Fat: 34.6g

Carbohydrate: 1.7g Net

Creamy Avocado Chiller with Twist of Lime

Total time: 4 hrs

Servings: 6

Ingredients:

□   Zest of 1 lime

□   Juice of 2 limes

□   2 large and ripe avocados

□   ½ cup erythritol

□   20 drops of stevia

□   2 cups coconut milk

Directions:

Peel the avocados and remove the seeds. Scoop out the flesh and mash them thoroughly in the food processor.

Now, add the coconut milk, lime zest, lime juice, erythritol and stevia and blend for a few more seconds to make a smooth paste.

Pour the paste into Popsicle molds and keep in fridge for about 4 hours.

Serve chilled.

Nutrition per Serving

Protein: 2.9g

Fat: 25.9g

Carbohydrate: 5.3g Ne

Choco-Avocado Fantasy Ice Cream

Total time: 1 hour

Servings: 8

Ingredients:

- 2 cups of coconut milk

- 1 tsp avocado extract

- 20 drops of stevia

- 2 large and ripe avocados

- ½ cup erythritol

- 1 tbsp peppermint extract

- 1 package of dark chocolate chips

Directions:

Smash the avocado flesh and blend with the coconut milk, mint, powdered erythritol and stevia with it. When a smooth paste is made, add the avocado extract and blend to get a really smooth paste.

Put the entire mixture into the ice cream maker and follow the instructions provided by the manufacturer to make the ice cream.

Serve chilled by garnishing with freshly chopped avocado and chocolate chips.

Nutrition per Serving

Protein: 3.6g

Fat: 25.3g

Carbohydrate: 5.7g Net

Majestic Tart with Avocado Flavored Curd

Total time: 2 hrs 30 mins

Servings: 8

Ingredients for making the crust:

- ☐ 4 large eggs

- ☐ ½ cup powdered erythritol

- ☐ 1 cup coconut flour

- ☐ ½ cup coconut oil

- ☐ 1 tsp avocado extract

Ingredients for making the avocado curd:

- ☐ Juice of ½ lemon

- ☐ 2 cups of mashed avocado flesh

- ☐ 1 tsp lemon zest

- ☐ ½ cup powdered erythritol

- ☐ 1 tbsp arrowroot powder

- ☐ 2 tbsp water

- ☐ 1 tbsp butter

- ☐ 20 drops of stevia

- ☐ 2 large egg yolks

Ingredients for topping:

☐   Lemon zest for garnishing

☐   1 cup chopped avocado

Directions:

To make the avocado curd, mix the mashed avocado with lemon juice, lemon zest, stevia, erythritol and water and bring the mixture to boil. Once it starts to boil, bring down the heat and simmer for the next 5 minutes. Then remove from heat and use a hand blender to make a smooth paste.

Keep the egg yolks ready and mix it with arrowroot powder. Add it to the avocado mixture and boil it over medium heat. Keep stirring to avoid burning at the bottom. As soon as the mixture starts bubbling, add butter and transfer the curd in a bowl. The bowl is to be covered with plastic so that a skin is not developed at the top. Keep in fridge for chilling.

Keep the oven ready by preheating at 300 degrees.

Make a mixture of eggs, coconut oil and avocado extract and then add the erythritol followed by coconut flour. The flour will absorb all moisture and make the batter thick.

Pour this batter into tart pans and press to give proper shape. Bake them for 10 minutes; make sure that the edges are brown. Take them out and allow cooling down.

Pour the curd filling with spoon and then top with lemon zest and chopped avocados.

Nutrition per Serving

Protein: 7g

Fat: 14.3g

Carbohydrate: 6.6g Net

Choco-Nutty Avocado Balls

Total time: 2 hrs

Servings: 25

Ingredients:

- ¼ cup coconut oil

- 125 dark chocolate

- 1 cup mashed avocado flesh

- 1½ cups chopped walnuts

- 1 tsp cinnamon

- 1 tbsp natural avocado extract

- 15 drops of stevia

Directions:

The chocolate is to be melted in hot water bath and then blend in the coconut oil, cinnamon and stevia. When the paste is smooth add the avocado extract and mashed avocado flesh along with chopped walnuts.

Pour this mixture into paper muffin cups and keep in fridge to harden. When they are semi-hard, bring out and roll between the palms to make balls and take them back to the fridge to chill.

Serve cold.

Nutrition per Serving

Protein: 1.5g

Fat: 8.4g

Carbohydrate: 1.5g Net

Interesting Candies with Avocado & Marshmallow

Total time: 35 mins

Servings: 4

Ingredients:

- ☐ 11 oz mashed avocado flesh

- ☐ 1/3 batch of low-carb marshmallows

- ☐ 1/3 cup butter

- ☐ 10 drops of stevia

Directions:

Mix the avocado flesh with butter and stevia.

Keep the marshmallows ready and top them with the avocado mixture and grill in oven for 10 minutes.

The candies can be served both warm and chilled.

Nutrition per Serving

Protein: 3.8g

Fat: 12.3g

Carbohydrate: 5.1g Net

Delightful Muffins with Bacon & Avocado

Total time: 30 mins

Servings: 16

Ingredients:

- ½ cup almond flour
- 2 tbsp butter
- 5 slices of bacon
- 5 large eggs
- 1½ tsp psyllium husk powder
- ¼ cup flaxseed meal
- 4.5 oz Colby Jack cheese
- 2 medium avocados, cut into cubes
- 1 tsp minced garlic
- 1 tsp dried chives
- Salt and pepper
- 3 medium spring onions
- 1 tsp dried cilantro
- 1 tsp baking powder
- 1½ tbsp lemon juice

☐　　¼ tsp red chilli flakes

☐　　1½ cup coconut milk (unsweetened)

Directions:

Put eggs, flaxseed, almond flour, psyllium husk powder, coconut milk and lemon juice in a bowl and blend them thoroughly. Keep the mixture aside.

Cook the bacon over medium heat to make them crisp and then add butter to the pan.

Now add the cubed avocados and add it to the bacon and cook for a minute.

Keep the oven ready by preheating at 350 degrees and then pour the batter into 16 muffin cups. Bake them for 26 minutes and make sure that they are golden in color. Allow cooling before taking out the muffins from the cups.

Serve after keeping in fridge for 15 minutes.

Nutrition per Serving

Protein: 6.1g

Fat: 14.1g

Carbohydrate: 1.5g Net

Avocado Muffin Delight with Pistachio Nuts

Total time: 40 mins

Servings: 8

Ingredients:

- 1 cup mashed avocado flesh

- 1½ cup almond flour

- ¼ cup coconut oil

- 2 large eggs

- ½ tsp apple cider vinegar

- ½ tsp ginger

- 3 bars of 90% chocolate

- ½ cup erythritol

- ½ cup pistachio nuts

- 2 tsp vanilla

- ½ tsp baking soda

- 1½ tsp cinnamon

- ½ tsp nutmeg

- ½ tsp cloves

Directions:

Preheat the oven at 325 degrees.

Use a large mixing bowl to blend almond flour with baking soda, erythritol and spices.

Use another bowl to mix the mashed avocado, coconut oil, large eggs, apple cider vinegar and vanilla. Now, blend the dry and wet mixtures thoroughly.

Chop the chocolate bars into smaller pieces and then add them along with the pistachio nuts to the batter. Use a spoon to distribute them evenly.

Divide the batter between 8 cupcake molds and bake them for 30 minutes. Make sure that the top of the muffins becomes golden brown in color.

Nutrition per Serving

Protein: 6.6g

Fat: 21.5g

Carbohydrate: 4g Net

Fruit & Nut Muffin Puncher with Twist of Chocolate

Total time: 15 mins

Servings: 12

Ingredients:

- 1 cup sunflower seed butter
- 1 ripe avocado
- ¼ cup chopped almonds
- 2 tbsp cocoa powder
- 6 tbsp water
- 2 large eggs
- ¼ cup chocolate chips
- ½ tsp avocado extract
- 1 tsp baking soda
- ¼ cup erythritol

Directions:

Preheat the oven at 350 degrees and grease 24 mini muffin tins.

Add the sunflower butter with avocado, eggs and water and use a hand blender to make smooth paste. Add cocoa powder, baking soda, erythritol and avocado extract to this mixture and blend again to get smooth batter.

Pour the batter into the mini muffin molds and top them with chocolate chips. Bake the muffins for 12 minutes and then allow standing for some time before taking them out from the molds.

Nutrition per Serving

Protein: 7g

Fat: 12.6g

Carbohydrate: 7.7g Ne

Pecan & Avocado Muffin Splendor

Total time: 30 mins

Servings: 12

Ingredients:

- ☐ 1 cup almond flour
- ☐ 1½ cups mashed avocado flesh
- ☐ ¾ cup erythritol
- ☐ 2 large eggs
- ☐ ½ cup softened butter
- ☐ 1 cup pecans, roughly chopped
- ☐ A pinch of salt
- ☐ 2.5 oz 90% chocolate
- ☐ 1 tbsp molasses

Directions:

Preheat the oven at 325 degrees and line the muffin tin with paper liners. Whisk erythritol with almond flour, pecans and salt and keep the mixture aside.

Use another bowl to beat the butter with eggs and molasses and then blend in the mixture of almond flour. It will be best to use a hand blender to make smooth batter.

Divide the batter into the muffin cups and bake them for 28 minutes. Allow cooling down before taking out from the molds.

Nutrition per Serving

Protein: 1.5g

Fat: 9.2g

Carbohydrate: 3.3g Net

Macadamia Magic Muffins with Bliss of Avocado

Total time: 35 mins

Servings: 12

Ingredients:

- 2 cups avocado flesh
- 3 cups of almond flour
- 1½ tsp baking powder
- 1 tsp baking soda
- ½ cup softened butter
- ½ tsp salt
- 1 tsp avocado extract
- 3 large eggs
- 20 drops of stevia extract
- ½ cup almond milk
- ½ cup erythritol
- 1/3 cup whey protein powder
- 8 tbsp chopped macadamia nuts

Directions:

Keep the oven ready by preheating at 325 degrees and then line the muffin tin with paper liners.

Mix protein powder, almond flour, baking soda, baking powder and salt and keep aside.

Use another bowl to beat the butter to make it smooth and then add erythritol, eggs, avocado extract and stevia. Now, blend the dry mixture with the wet one very slowly, pouring the almond milk in between. Reserve 2 tablespoons of chopped nuts for garnishing and add the rest into the batter. Use a spoon to distribute them evenly.

Pour the batter into the muffin cups and then top each muffin with chopped nuts.

Bake them for 30 minutes, make sure that the muffins are golden in color and then allow enough time to cool down.

Nutrition per Serving

Protein: 6g

Fat: 7.9g

Carbohydrate: 5.5g Net

Spicy Avocado Muffins with Blissful Orange Glaze

Total time: 32 mins

Servings: 10

Ingredients for making the spicy avocado muffins:

- ¼ cup granulated erythritol

- ¼ cup whey protein powder

- ½ tsp baking soda

- 2 cups of almond flour

- 1 tbsp garam masala

- 2 tsp baking powder

- 4 oz cream cheese

- ½ tsp salt

- 2 large eggs

- ¼ cup butter

- 24 drops of stevia extract

- ¼ cup almond milk

- Ingredients for making orange glaze:

☐ 1 tbsp orange juice

☐ ¼ cup powdered erythritol

Directions:

Preheat the oven at 325 degrees and line the muffin cups with paper liners.

Blend the wet and dry ingredients separately and then mix them together to form the muffin batter.

Pour the batter into the muffin cups and bake them for 27 minutes. Make sure that they are golden in color.

Make the orange glaze by mixing the erythritol with the orange juice and then drizzle over the muffins.

Nutrition per Serving

Protein: 3.9g

Fat: 2g

Carbohydrate: 3.9g Net

Exclusive Avocado & Cranberry Muffins

Total time: 20 mins

Servings: 12

Ingredients:

- ½ cup flax seed meal
- 1½ cup mashed avocado flesh
- ½ tsp xanthan gum
- 1/2 cup butter
- 1/3 cup erythritol
- 2 tsp baking powder
- 3 eggs
- ½ tsp salt
- 1/3 cup water
- 1 cup whole cranberries
- 1/3 cup water

Directions:

Keep the oven ready by preheating at 350 degrees and line the muffin cups with paper liners.

Make a mixture with flax seed meal, xanthan gum, baking powder and salt.

Add the butter, eggs and water to this mixture and beat thoroughly to make the muffin batter. Finally stir in the cranberries.

Pour the batter into muffin cups and bake them for 15 minutes, making sure that the top is well set.

Allow complete cooling and then serve.

Nutrition per Serving

Protein: 3.9g

Fat: 8g

Carbohydrate: 1.6g Net

Lemon & Avocado Tart (without baking)

Total time: 15 mins

Servings: 24

Ingredients for making the crust:

☐   ¾ cup dried coconut (finely grated)

☐   3 tbsp lemon juice

☐   Pinch of salt

☐   1½ tsp vanilla extract

- ☐ 2 tbsp erythritol

- ☐ 4½ tbsp butter

Ingredients for making the avocado filling:

- ☐ 1/3 cup full fat coconut milk

- ☐ 1 tsp vanilla extract

- ☐ ¼ tsp salt

- ☐ Zest of 2 medium lemons

- ☐ ½ cup butter

- ☐ 2 tsp lemon extract

- ☐ 1 cup mashed avocado flesh

- ☐ 1 tbsp erythritol

Directions:

Grease 24 mini-muffin cups and keep them aside.

Put all the tart making ingredients in a large mixing bowl. Blend them thoroughly to make tight dough and then roll the dough to form a big roll. Now, cut the dough into 24 equal parts and press each into the one muffin cup. Keep in fridge to chill.

To make the avocado filling, beat the butter till it becomes fluffy and then add coconut milk, erythritol, vanilla and lemon extract, lemon zest and salt and beat to make a smooth mixture.

Spoon the filling mixture into each chilled crust and return them back to fridge so that they can set.

Nutrition per Serving

Protein: 1.3g

Fat: 10.3g

Carbohydrate: 2.18g Net

Super Easy Avocado Guacamole Balls

Total time; 45 mins

Servings: 6

Ingredients:

- ½ large avocado

- ¼ cup butter

- 1 small chilli pepper

- 2 cloves of crushed garlic

- ¼ tsp salt

- Ground black pepper, according to taste

- 1 tbsp fresh lime juice

- ½ small white onion

- 4 slices of bacon

Directions:

Keep the oven ready by preheating at 375 degrees and line a baking tray with baking paper.

Lay the bacon strips on the tray and cook in oven for 15 minutes, ensuring they become golden brown and then keep them aside. Prepare the avocado by peeling and deseeding and then keep it in a bowl along with chilli pepper, butter, lime juice and garlic.

Use a potato masher to make a smooth paste with the mentioned ingredients and then add the onion before final mixing. Make sure to add the bacon grease from the baking tray. Keep the mixture in fridge for 20 minutes and then take them out to make small balls from the mixture.

Crumble the cooked bacon and then roll the guacamole balls over the bacon crumbs.

Keep in fridge and then serve chilled.

Nutrition per Serving

Protein: 3.4g

Fat: 15.2g

Carbohydrate: 1.4g Net

Magical Avocado Filled Candy

Total time: 45 mins

Servings: 24

Ingredients for the coating:

- ☐ 2/3 cup Swerve confectioners

- ☐ 1 tsp lemon extract

- ☐ 4 oz cocoa butter

- ☐ ¼ tsp Celtic sea salt

Ingredients for the avocado filling:

- ☐ ½ cup lemon juice

- ☐ 1 cup erythritol

- ☐ 1 large avocado, only flesh

- ☐ 1 tbsp finely grated lemon peel

- ☐ 4 large eggs

- ☐ 8 tbsp coconut oil

Directions:

Melt the cocoa butter in a double boiler and then add the lemon extract along with sweetener and salt. Pour the mixture into truffle mold and place in fridge to become solid.

Make the lemon filling by mixing the sweetener with lemon juice, eggs, avocado flesh, and lemon peel in a medium skillet over medium heat. Once properly mixed, keep the mixture in cold bath for 15 minutes.

Pour the cooled down filling into the truffle mold and then top the open end with more cocoa butter mixture. Put them back in the fridge to solidify and serve chilled.

Nutrition per Serving

Protein: 1.1g

Fat: 10.g

Carbohydrate: 0.2g Net

Easiest Ever Avocado Fat Bombs

Total time: 1 hr

Servings: 16

Ingredients:

- ¼ cup coconut oil

- 7.1 oz coconut butter

- 1½ cups avocado flesh, mashed

- Pinch of salt

- 20 drops of stevia

Directions:

Put avocado flesh in the food processor and then run the device to make puree of the fruit. Now, add coconut oil and coconut butter. Blend in all the other ingredients together and then pour them in mini-muffin cups.

Keep them in the fridge for 50 minutes and then serve chilled.

Nutrition per Serving

Protein: 0.76g

Fat: 11.9g

Carbohydrate: 0.8g Net

Avocado & Cacao Butter Fat Booster

Total time: 10 mins

Servings: 24

Ingredients:

- [ ] 10 oz coconut milk
- [ ] 2 cups avocado flesh
- [ ] 6 oz cacao butter
- [ ] ½ cup coconut oil
- [ ] 1 tsp avocado extract
- [ ] A pinch of salt
- [ ] ½ cup vanilla protein powder
- [ ] 1 tsp liquid stevia
- [ ] ½ cup thinly sliced avocados

Directions:

Use a sauce pan to melt the cacao butter over low heat and then blend in the coconut milk and coconut oil. Now, whisk in the protein powder, avocado extract, stevia and salt only after turning off the heat and then pour the mixture on a parchment paper.

Sprinkle the avocado slices on top and keep it in the fridge for a couple of hours.

Cut into 24 slices and serve.

Nutrition per Serving

Protein: 2.2g

Fat: 17.8g

Carbohydrate: 1.2g Net

Blackberry & Avocado Fat Enhancer

Total time: 10 mins

Servings: 16

Ingredients:

☐ 1 cup coconut oil

☐ 1 cup almond butter

☐ 1 cup mashed avocado flesh

☐ ¼ tsp liquid stevia

☐ ¼ tsp vanilla powder

☐ 1 tsp lemon juice

☐ ½ cup fresh blackberries

Directions:

Keep the blackberries with almond butter and coconut oil in a pot and heat them over medium heat. Add the remaining ingredients and use a hand blender to make smooth paste and spread it out the paste on a baking tray lined with parchment paper.

Keep it in the fridge for some time and when it becomes solid, cut into serving size squares.

Nutrition per Serving

Protein: 1.3g

Fat: 18.7g

Carbohydrate: 2g Net

Chocolate Rich Nutty Avocado Fat Blast

Total time: 15 mins

Servings: 6

Ingredients:

- 2 tbsp unsweetened cocoa powder

- 2 oz cocoa butter

- 2 tbsp Swerve

- ¼ cup heavy cream

- 4 oz chopped pistachio nuts

- 1½ cups mashed avocado flesh

Directions:

Melt the cocoa butter in a double boiler and then put it in a sauce pan.

Add cocoa powder to it and then add the Swerve along with the pistachio nuts followed by the cream and mashed avocado flesh.

Pour the mixture into mini-muffin cups and then keep them in fridge so that they can set well. Serve chilled.

Nutrition per Serving

Protein: 3g

Fat: 28g

Carbohydrate: 3g Net

Fat Bars with Avocado, Almonds & Coconut

Total time: 20 mins

Servings: 5

Ingredients:

- 1 cup unsweetened coconut, shredded
- 1 cup mashed avocado flesh
- 1 packet of stevia
- 1+ ½   teaspoon avocado extract
- 2 oz + 4 tbsp coconut oil (for coating)
- 4 tbsp roasted almonds, finely chopped
- ⅓ cup coconut cream

Directions:

Put the shredded coconut, coconut cream and avocado in a bowl and use a spoon to mix it thoroughly.

Pour a spoonful of the mixture on a parchment paper lined cookie sheet and make use of a spatula to make rectangular shaped bars. Keep them in fridge for a couple of hours.

Make the avocado coating by melting the coconut oil and adding the avocado extract along with the avocado extract and stevia. Stir well so that all the ingredients are properly incorporated and then let it cool down at room temperature.

Bring out the bars and dip each one in the avocado mixture and take the coated bars to the fridge so that the coating is properly set.

Nutrition per Serving

Protein: 1g

Fat: 22g

Carbohydrate: 4.8g

Cheesy Avocado Magical Blaster

Total time: 5 hours

Servings: 16

Ingredients

- ☐ 4 tbsp butter

- ☐ 2 cups mashed avocado flesh

- ☐ 1 tsp avocado extract

- ☐ 4 tbsp virgin coconut oil

- ☐ 2oz cream cheese

- ☐ 4 tbsp heavy cream

- ☐ Sweetener to taste

Directions:

Heat the heavy cream in a pan and keep it aside.

Heat the butter and coconut oil in a pan and then blend it with heavy cream. Whisk them thoroughly to get a smooth paste.

Mash the avocado flesh once again and add the sweetener. Blend it with the buttery mixture and pour the final mixture into muffin cups.

Keep in fridge overnight and serve chilled.

Nutrition per Serving

Protein: 0.4 g

Fat: 8.1 g

Carbohydrate: 0.8 g